T5-AVO-819

DISCARDED BY

MACPHÁIDÍN LIBRARY

CUSHING-MARTIN LIBRARY
STONEHILL COLLEGE
NORTH EASTON, MASSACHUSETTS

RB
155
E83

The Etiology of
Inherited Disorders

Papers by
C. B. Kerr, Donald L. Rucknagel, R. E.
Brown et al.

102288

MSS Information Corporation
655 Madison Avenue, New York, N.Y. 10021

Library of Congress Cataloging in Publication Data
Main entry under title:

Etiology of inherited disorders.

   1. Medical genetics--Addresses, essays, lectures.
I. Kerr, Charles Baldwin, 1932-   [DNLM: 1. Heredi-
tary diseases--Etiology--Collected works. QZ50 E85 1973]
RB155.E83   616'.042   73-11118
ISBN 0-8422-7151-1

Copyright © 1974
by MSS Information Corporation
All Rights Reserved

TABLE OF CONTENTS

CREDITS AND ACKNOWLEDGEMENTS

Brown, R.E.; P.J.S. Hamilton; J. Kagwa; and M.A. Warley, "Is Marriage Counseling Feasible in Africa to Prevent Sickle-Cell Disease?," *Clinical Pediatrics*, 1969, 8:421-424.

Campbell, Maurice, "Common Malformations of the Heart," *Guy's Hospital Reports*, 1967, 116:341-349.

Goldschmidt, Ernst, "Experiences from 5 Years of Genetic Counseling in Eye Diseases," *Acta Ophthalmologica*, 1968, 46:463-468.

Jaworska, Mieczylawa; and Jerzy Popiolek, "Genetic Counselling in Lobster-Claw Anomaly: Discussion of Variability of Genetic Influence in Different Families," *Clinical Pediatrics*, 1968, 7:396-399.

Kerr, C.B., "Genetic Counseling in Hereditary Disorders of Blood Coagulation," *Modern Treatment*, 1968, 5:125-133.

Lowry, R.B.; J.A. Birbeck; P.H. Padwick; and Betty J. Wood, "Cartilage-Hair Hypoplasia: A Rare and Recessive Cause of Dwarfism," *Clinical Pediatrics*, 1970, 9:44-46.

Lynch, Henry T., "Practical Aspects of the Family History, Genetics, and Genetics Counseling: Cancer," *Nebraska State Medical Journal*, 1968, 53:6-11.

Lynch, Henry T.; and Anne J. Krush, "Genetic Counseling and Cancer Control," *Southern Medical Journal*, 1968, 61:265-269.

Nora, James J.; Paul F. Dodd; Dan G. McNamara; Michael A.W. Hattwick; Robert D. Leachman; and Denton A. Cooley, "Risk to Offspring of Parents with Congenital Heart Defects," *Journal of the American Medical Association*, 1969, 209:2052-2053.

Rogers, Blair O., "Microtic, Lop, Cup and Protruding Ears: Four Directly Inheritable Deformities?," *Plastic and Reconstructive Surgery*, 1968, 41:208-231.

Rucknagel, Donald L.; and Russel K. Laros, "Hemoglobinopathies: Genetics and Implications for Studies of Human Reproduction," *Clinical Obstetrics and Gynecology*, 1969, 12:49-75.

Shannon, Michael W.; and Henry L. Nadler, "X-Linked Hydrocephalus," *Journal of Medical Genetics*, 1968, 5:326-328.

Whelan, Donald T.; and Charles R. Scriver, "Cystathioninuria and Renal Iminoglycinuria in a Pedigree," *New England Journal of Medicine*, 1968, 278:924-927.

Zaremba, J., "Tuberous Sclerosis: A Clinical and Genetical Investigation," *Journal of Mental Deficiency Research*, 1968, 12:63-80.

PREFACE

According to one contributing author of this volume, "those who need advice on genetic risks need it badly. Decisions on planning a family and even on entering into marriage await the result of counseling." Old wives tales, anxiety, and guilt on the part of the individuals involved also complicate the clinical picture surrounding genetic counseling. Its goals in furthering an understanding of inherited disorders are explored in this new volume.

The most current research findings on the etiology of inherited human disorders, ranging from hemoglobinopathies to cartilage-hair hypoplasia, are covered. Diseases such as cancer and heart defects are viewed from a genetic perspective, and early diagnosis of certain types of cancer is tentatively linked to genetic heritage.

Genetic Counseling in Hereditary Disorders of Blood Coagulation

C. B. KERR, M.B., Ph.D.

THOSE WHO NEED ADVICE ON GENETIC RISKS need it badly. Decisions on planning a family and even on entering into marriage await the results of counseling. Inherited disease arouses strong emotions and frequently the situation is complicated by anxiety and guilt or confused by ignorance and old wives' tales. With so much at stake, genetic counseling must be regarded as an important component in over-all management.

With inherited disorders of blood coagulation, the fundamental requirements for counseling are a detailed family history and full facilities for investigating hemostatic mechanisms, together with a knowledge of patterns of inheritance and the manner in which each mutation expresses its effect in the individual.

In practice, by far the most frequent requests for counseling come from female relatives of males with the sex-linked conditions of classic hemophilia (Factor VIII deficiency) and Christmas disease (Factor IX deficiency). With the exception of autosomal dominant inheritance in von Willebrand's disease (and a few unique conditions) almost all other coagulation disorders are autosomal recessive conditions. A deficiency of fibrin-stabilizing factor (Factor XIII) may possibly be inherited in two ways—as an autosomal recessive trait and as a sex-linked characteristic (15). A detailed account of genetic aspects has been given elsewhere (6).

RECESSIVE DISORDERS

Autosomal recessive inheritance is found in hereditary deficiencies of fibrinogen (Factor I), prothrombin (Factor II), proaccelerin (Factor V), Factor VII, Stuart factor (Factor X), plasma thromboplastin antecedent (Factor XI), Hageman factor (Factor XII), and fibrin-stabilizing factor (Factor XIII). These are extremely rare conditions with population frequencies of 1×10^{-5} to 10^{-6}. A possible exception is PTA deficiency, which has been reported almost solely in Jews and is not infrequent among the Jewish community of New York (18).

The usual situation for counseling is that clinically normal heterozygous parents, each carrying the mutant gene, have given birth to an affected homozygous child and wish to know the risks to further offspring. For each subsequent conception, the risk that the disease will recur will be 1 in 4. If the affected child, in turn, has offspring, the chances that any will be affected are negligible, because it is highly improbable that an unrelated marriage partner from the general population would carry the same rare gene. The exceptional situation with recessive conditions is, of course, marriage of a heterozygous carrier to a blood relative, most usually a cousin. This is because carriers share genes derived from the common ancestor; in the case of first cousin partners, 12.5 per cent of all genes are common to both. Looked at in another way, consanguineous marriages are over-represented among the parents of children with rare recessive disorders. Rather less than 1 per cent of all marriages in Western countries are between related persons. By contrast, it was found that parents were cousins in 43 per cent of recorded families with afibrinogenemia, 50 per cent of those deficient in fibrin-stabilizing factor, and 30 per cent of those with a deficiency of proaccelerin (6).

The question of consanguinity arises not only with regard to cousins from families at risk but also in inbred communities, such as Jewish people in New York (with regard to PTA deficiency) and geographically isolated communities containing families like those reported from Switzerland in which the genes for Stuart factor or fibrin-stabilizing factor deficiencies were segregating.

Tests for the detection of carriers become relevant in such situations, and semiquantitative assays are available for measuring the concentrations of the pertinent factors in all autosomal recessive disorders. If a level intermediate between zero and the average normal concentration is found under carefully controlled conditions, it can be taken as evidence of the carrier state. Such is the case for deficiencies of proaccelerin, Stuart factor, PTA, Hageman factor, and fibrin-stabilizing factor, but not in afibrinogenemia (11,14) or Factor VII deficiency (9), where a proportion of known carriers has normal factor levels as measured by current methods. In the absence of unequivocal laboratory evidence of heterozygosity, the alternative is to calculate the risk on the basis of Mendelian theory. For instance, if a known carrier marries a first cousin of unknown genetic status, the chances are 1 in 8 that the latter carries the same mutant gene and so the *a priori* risk of having an affected child is 1 in 32.

DOMINANT CONDITIONS

Excluding unique and vague disorders (reviewed in detail elsewhere (6)), von Willebrand's disease is the only condition of practical significance with autosomal dominant inheritance. Typically, affected members are found in each generation and affected children have one or the other parent with the disease.

The most frequent indications for counseling involve estimating the risk to children of an affected parent and ascertaining whether or not a relative of a patient carries the mutant gene. And a critical point in evaluation is the variable expression of gene effect in von Willebrand's disease. Expression may be considered in terms of clinical severity, and ranges from the absence of hemorrhagic symptoms to seriously impaired hemostasis. In addition, it is often said that the gene has variable penetrance, implying that in a group of persons known from pedigree evidence to possess the mutation, there are some with no detectable sign of its effects. This is true at a clinical level, but is not so certain in terms of laboratory measures because of the varying precision of different techniques. For instance, the Duke method of recording the bleeding time is far less reliable than the Ivy technique (12).

It follows that counseling has to take into account the consequences of varying expressivity. The risk that an offspring of an affected parent will have the disease is 1 in 2. If, however, the parent displays only a mild form of the disorder, this does not imply necessarily that a child will be affected to a similar minor degree; the chances are at least 50 per cent that the child will have significant hemostatic problems. And, of course, the reverse situation holds; a severely affected parent can have a mildly affected child.

The question of nonpenetrance (or zero expressivity) arises when a clinically normal relative of an individual with proven von Willebrand's disease wishes to know about the risks to his children. If such a person is at genetic risk himself, if for example, he is the child of an affected parent, and careful laboratory investigations are entirely normal, then it is probably wise to allow for a slight degree of nonpenetrance. There is nothing to suggest that the latter would exceed 10 per cent, and so the advice in this situation would incorporate a relatively slight risk, about 1 in 20, of carrying the gene. This would give a risk to each offspring of 1 in 40.

11

Von Willebrand's disease varies in frequency. About 10 per cent of Åland islanders in the Baltic are affected, but the usual rate of case detection is in the order of $1-2 \times 10^{-5}$. Presumptive homozygotes have been described; some appear to have a more extreme hemorrhagic disease (4).

There is no indication of the mutation rate in von Willebrand's disease, but isolated cases do occur, and because the genetic situation is so different from that in classic hemophilia it is important to exclude the possibility of von Willebrand's disease in any male with a moderate or mild deficiency of antihemophilic factor.

SEX-LINKED CONDITIONS

Identical genetic principles apply to both classic hemophilia and Christmas disease. Together, these conditions account for over 95 per cent of all persons with an isolated clotting factor deficiency. The prevalence of affected males in a Western community is around 1 per 10,000 total males, with a deficiency of antihemophilic factor being encountered 4 times as frequently as that of Christmas factor.

The outstanding feature of sex-linked inheritance is that no affected male can transmit his X-chromosome and hence the mutant gene to his son. When the sex-linked gene is recessive or incompletely recessive, as in the conditions under discussion, significant bleeding symptoms in carriers are quite exceptional.

The most frequent request for counseling comes from women in hemophilic families. Certain women are definite carriers. Daughters of affected men *must* have the gene because all receive their father's single X-chromosome. Similarly, women with an affected son and another hemophilic relative in the maternal line must be carriers. The same principles apply to Christmas disease.

Definite carriers will have, on the average, half of their sons affected; the risk to infants at each conception is 1 in 4. Hemophilic men can be informed that the grandsons born to their daughters stand a 50 per cent chance of being affected. An exception occurs when a hemophiliac marries a cousin who is a carrier (5 instances are on record (6)). In this type of union, there is a 50 per cent risk to sons, and daughters have an equal chance of being either affected homozygotes, that is, true hemophiliacs, or heterozygotes.

Most commonly, women who seek advice are those with a 50 per cent or lesser risk of being a carrier. These are the sisters of hemophiliacs, mothers of a bleeder with no family history of hemophilia, or a more distantly related woman in the maternal line. The *a priori* probability of heterozygosity can be calculated in each case; for distant relatives, a mathematical study is available (1). With a serious illness such as the severe form of hemophilia, however, even giving fairly long odds on the chances of heterozygosity, say 1 in 20, may be quite unsatisfactory to a woman at risk. Such women require a definite answer, and the only solution is through laboratory identification of the carrier state.

Claims on the percentage of known carriers that can be detected by a reduced plasma concentration of antihemophilic factor range from zero (3) to 94 per cent (13). The current consensus (7,8), however, is that a group of carriers will have a distribution of antihemophilic factor values with a mean of 50 per cent of the average-normal concentration, one which overlaps the distribution in normal females. But there is no doubt that a proportion of carriers can be identified by the fact that the concentration of antihemophilic factor in their plasma values is significantly reduced below normal—perhaps 2–2.5 standard deviations below the normal mean.

It is, of course, necessary when investigating women at risk, to avoid situations known to elevate the concentration of antihemophilic factor; for instance, exercise, pregnancy, and recent trauma. Statistical analyses of laboratory data with regard to carrier detection have been described in detail (7,16).

Women with unequivocably low concentrations of antihemophilic factor can be told that they are carriers, but it follows from what has been described above that *a concentration within normal limits does not exclude the possibility of heterozygosity.* The latter situation may arise in a woman with an affected son and no family history of hemophilia. A fresh mutation must account for a proportion of such cases. For counseling purposes it is important to know where the mutation occurred. If it originated in an X-chromosome of the maternal ovum destined to form the first affected son, the chances of a second mutation occurring in a subsequent ovum are very slight, because of the over-all rarity of such genetic disturbances. Unfortunately, nothing is known about the origin of mutations, although some indirect evidence has been interpreted as indicating that the event occurs most frequently in the X-chromosome contributed by the father of a woman with a single affected child (2). At present, it must be accepted that the mother of a sporadic hemophiliac has a fairly high risk of having another affected male. Assuming an equal probability of a mutation occurring in a grand-paternal sperm, grand-maternal ovum, and maternal ovum, the risk to any subsequent son would be 1 in 6. If the sperm is indeed more frequently involved the risk will be greater than 1 in 6.

It has been suggested that comparison of antihemophilic factor concentrations in carriers and their normal brothers demonstrated differences that were sufficiently great to be of value in the detection of carriers (10). This observation has not been confirmed (7,19), and neither have other intrafamilial comparisons proved to be of practical significance (8). At one time it was thought that carriers of mild antihemophilic factor deficiency had a consistently greater reduction in the concentration of this factor than carriers of the severe variety (5). This distinction was subsequently proved invalid (6,7).

What has been stated above for classic hemophilia applies equally to Christmas disease. Males with either condition who are related to one another have similar laboratory and clinical findings; it is quite exceptional to find bleeders of varying severity in the same family. This point may require emphasis when counseling; there is nothing to suggest that a mildly affected male will be born in a family with severe hemophilia or Christmas disease, or vice versa.

It appears unlikely that the present unsatisfactory state of carrier detection will be resolved by the construction of more refined assay methods for plasma antihemophilic factor or Christmas factor. In fact, a solution for all cases may not be possible until the synthesis of clotting factors can be examined at a cellular level. If Lyon's inactive X-chromosome theory applies to sex-linked coagulation disorders, there is a theoretic possibility of finding in carriers a mosaic cell population with regard to the synthesis of these two factors (8).

Females who have the full clinical and laboratory features of hemophilia are rare, but over 60 well-documented cases are on record. Observed and postulated mechanisms are:

1. Homozygosity resulting from the union of an affected male with a carrier female.
2. Extreme expression in a female of the usually recessive sex-linked mutation.
3. Discordant or abnormal sex chromosome complements so that the affected female has the male XY pattern, as in testicular feminization, or an XO karyotype, as in Turner's syndrome.
4. Misdiagnosis of von Willebrand's disease.
5. A proportion of sporadic cases, in males and females, may result from homozygosity for an autosomal mutation, which yields a phenotype indistinguishable from that for the X-linked variety.

Little is known about the group of patients with fibrin-stabilizing factor deficiency who may possibly inherit their defect via an abnormality of the X-chromosome. Presumably, such individuals will have genetic problems similar to those in classic hemophilia and Christmas disease.

SOME ADDITIONAL SITUATIONS

The aim of genetic counseling is to give advice that will assist members of a family in making decisions. There are no scientific or moral grounds for qualifying such advice with personal views on the acceptability of a given risk. Admittedly, some persons do require help in planning courses of action, and the logical choice of an advisor is a physician with considerable knowledge of the family. Sometimes, experts in other fields may be needed. For instance, certain situations in hemophilia may conflict with religious teachings on such matters as transfusion of blood, ritual circumcision, or contraception.

For known or possible carriers of hemophilia, a policy of permitting the birth of females and aborting males was proposed by Danish workers (17). They made antenatal determinations of fetal sex by analyzing the sex chromatin of amniotic cells obtained by uterine puncture during the third trimester. There are many problems inherent in this policy, including those of a legal, psychologic, and cytodiagnostic nature.

An important corollary of counseling is to assist in assuaging guilt feelings. This is particularly relevant for female carriers of sex-linked diseases and the mothers of patients with sporadic disease. Tactless emphasis on the maternal side of the family when investigating and recording the pedigree of the disorder may tend to increase the mother's self-incriminatory tendency. Additional misconceptions about the mechanism of inheritance or psychic denial mechanisms often cloud the true genetic situation. Normal relatives who are not at risk may nevertheless feel uncertain about their children's future. In this instance the only solution in counseling is to offer a careful explanation of the pattern of inheritance and the lottery-like nature of fresh mutation.

Finally, it must be emphasized that genetic counseling has nothing to do with eugenics. The latter implies the promotion of policies which incorporate some measure of reducing the population frequency of harmful genes and which generally involve birth control, sterilization, and abortion. Apart from exceeding the confines of the physician-patient relationship, the results of such policies can be shown to have little advantage over conventional methods of counseling in a disease like hemophilia which is maintained in a population by an appreciable rate of mutation.

References

1. BINET, F. E., SAWERS, R. J., and WATSON, G. S.   Hereditary counseling for sex-linked recessive deficiency diseases. *Ann. hum. Genet.* 22:144, 1958.

2. BITTER, K.   Erhebungen zur Bestimmung der Mutationsrate für Haemophilie A und B in Hamburg. *Z. menschl. Vererb. Konstit. Lehre.* 37:251, 1963.

3. GARDIKAS, C., KATSIROUMBAS, P., and KOTTAS, C.   The antihaemophilic globulin concentration in the plasma of female carriers of haemophilia. *Brit. J. Haemat.* 3:377, 1957.

4. GRAHAM, J. B., BARROW, E. M., and ROBERTS, H. R.   "Possible Implications of the Autosomal and X-Linked Hemophilia Phenotypes." In *Genetics and the Interactions of Blood Clotting Factors.* Schattauer, Stuttgart, 1965.

5. GRAHAM, J. B., McLENDON, W. W., and BRINKHOUS, K. M.   Mild hemophilia: an allelic form of the disease. *Amer. J. Med. Sci.* 225:46, 1953.

6. KERR, C. B.   Genetics of human blood coagulation. *J. Med. Genet.* 2:221, 1965.

7. KERR, C. B., PRESTON, A. E., BARR, A., and BIGGS, R.   Further studies on the inheritance of Factor VIII. *Brit. J. Haemat.* 12:212, 1966.

8. KERR, C. B.   "The Detection of Carriers of Haemophilia." In *Proc. Symp. Haemophilia.* World Fed. Haemophilia, Sydney, 1966.

9. MARDER, V. J., and SHULMAN, N. R.   Clinical aspects of congenital Factor VII deficiency. *Amer. J. Med.* 37:182, 1964.

10. MULDER, E., MOCHTAR, I. A., VAN CREVELD, S., and LOPES-CARDOZA, E. B.   Factor VIII activity in carriers of Haemophilia A. *Brit. J. Haemat.* 11:206, 1965.

11. NIEWIAROWSKI, S., KOZLOWSKA, J., GULMANTOWICZ, A., and PELCZARSKA-KASPERKA, E.   Afibrinogénémie congénitale. *Hemostase.* 2:191, 1962.

12. NILSSON, I. M., MAGNUSSON, S., and BORCHGREVINK, C. F.   The Duke and Ivy methods for determination of the bleeding time. *Thrombos. Diathes. Haemorrh.* (Stuttg.) 10:223, 1963.

13. NILSSON, I. M., BLOMBÄCK, M., RAMGREN, O., and VON FRANCKEN, I.   Haemophilia in Sweden. II. Carriers of Haemophilia A and B. *Acta Med. Scand.* 171:223, 1962.

14. OSEID, S., and SVENDSEN, H. M.   Congenital afibrinogenemia. *Acta paediat.* 52:129, 1963.

15. PRENTICE, C. R. M., and RATNOFF, O. D.   Genetic disorders of blood coagulation. *Seminars in Hematology* 4:93, 1967.

16. RAPAPORT, S. I., PATCH, M. J., and MOORE, E. J.   Antihemophilic globulin levels in carriers of Hemophilia A. *J. Clin. Invest.* 39:1619, 1960.

17. Riis, P., and Fuchs, F. Antenatal determination of foetal sex in prevention of hereditary diseases. *Lancet* 2:180, 1960.

18. Rosenthal, R. L. Hemorrhage in PTA (Factor XI) deficiency (Abstr.). *Proc. Xth Cong. Internat. Soc. Haemat.* Stockholm, 1964.

19. Veltkamp, J. J., Hemker, H. L., and Loeliger, E. A. "Detection of Heterozygotes for Factors VIII, IX and XII Deficiency." In *Genetics and the Interaction of Blood Clotting Factors.* Schattauer, Stuttgart, 1965.

HEMOGLOBINOPATHIES: GENETICS AND IMPLICATIONS FOR STUDIES OF HUMAN REPRODUCTION

DONALD L. RUCKNAGEL, M.D., Ph.D., and
RUSSELL K. LAROS, Jr., M.D.

THE MODERN CONCEPT OF MOLECULAR GENETICS has unfolded rather rapidly in the short span of 2 decades, due in large measure to the conceptual contributions resulting from studies of the abnormal human hemoglobins, and in particular sickle cell anemia. From these studies the concept of the structural gene has emerged, in which genetic information is encoded in nuclear deoxyribonucleic acid such that each triplet of purine-pyrimidine base pairs constitutes a code word or *codon* equivalent to an amino acid residue in the polypeptide chain of proteins. This information is transcribed, as the process is designated, onto messenger ribonucleic acid, which in turn communicates the information from the nucleus to the cell's synthetic machinery in the cytoplasm. On the ribosomes the messenger RNA serves as a template for translating the genetic code into the protein gene product.

In addition to determining protein structure, other specialized genes control the rate at which proteins are synthesized—the so-called operator and regulator genes (for review see Watson). Although the concept of regulation has been formulated as a result of biochemical genetic studies of microorganisms, the thalassemia syndromes, which are related to the hemoglobinopathies, may be abberations in the human equivalent.

We will review here the genetic and molecular biochemistry of the hemoglobinopathies and thalassemia syndromes. In addition we will consider selected aspects of population genetics, the influence of hemoglobinopathies on human reproduction, and genetic counselling.

Supported in part by United States Public Health Service Grants 5-K3-GM-15,325, PO1-GM-15,419, and T12 CA 08098 from the National Institutes of Health.

19

Structural Genes

Although hemoglobin has been studied for over 100 years and is one of the most thoroughly characterized proteins, that aspect of its chemistry which is of most importance to the geneticist (7,12,13,23) is of relatively recent origin and evolved initially from interest in sickle cell anemia. In the interval from its description by Herrick in 1910, to 1949, the difference between the severe sickle cell anemia and the asymptomatic, nonanemic, sickle cell trait became appreciated. The relationship between the sickling phenomenon and oxygen tension also was delineated (references in Harris). In 1949 Neel and Beet demonstrated independently that both parents of children with sickle cell anemia had sickle cell trait and that the Mendelian 1:2:1 ratio obtained among the children (Fig. 1). In that

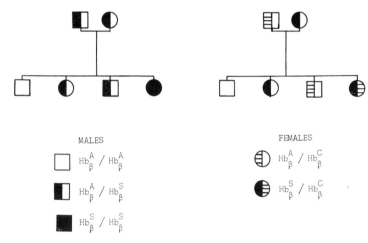

Fig. 1. *Left,* Mendelian genetics of sickle cell anemia, and *Right,* sickle cell-hemoglobin C disease, showing the segregation of alleles at $\underline{Hb_\beta}$ structural locus.

same year Pauling *et al.* demonstrated that all the hemoglobin of patients with sickle cell anemia and approximately one-half of that of persons with sickle cell trait migrated abnormally by moving boundary electrophoresis. Electrophoretic patterns using the newer cellulose acetate membranes are shown in Figure 2. Whereas the former observation showed clearly that sickle cell anemia is inherited and the latter that it is a "molecular" disease, the two observations

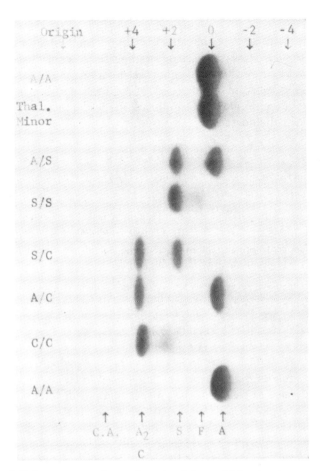

Fig. 2. Cellulose acetate electrophoresis of hemoglobin showing most common phenotypes. Two samples were applied to the left end of each 1″ × 6″ strip and electrophoresed in tris-borate-EDTA buffer at pH 8.6 and stained with ponceau S; the anode is on the right. Numbers at the top indicate net ionic charge relative to that of Hb A. The component migrating anodal to Hb C in the C/C specimen is a storage artifact. C.A. is carbonic anhydrase enzyme.

taken together implied that genes have something to do with protein structure.

POLYPEPTIDE CHAIN ALTERATIONS

The structural abnormality was clarified in 1956 when Ingram, using the peptide mapping or "fingerprinting" technique, showed that in hemoglobin's beta polypeptide chain a glutamic acid residue, now known to be the sixth from the free amino terminal end of the molecule, was replaced by a valine residue (Fig. 3). Since the side chain of glutamic acid may be negatively charged and that of valine is neutral, it follows that the charge of the Hb-S molecule is positive with respect to Hb A, thus explaining the differences in electrophoretic mobility. This substitution alters the physicochemical properties of the hemoglobin molecule which in turn leads to the protean manifestations of sickle cell anemia.

		Net charge difference
HbS	Val-His-Leu-Thre-Pro-Val-Glu-Lys	+1
HbA	Val-His-Leu-Thre-Pro-Glu-Glu-Lys	0
HbC	Val-His-Leu-Thre-Pro-Lys-Glu-Lys	+2

Fig. 3. **Amino acid sequence of the first tryptic peptide of hemoglobin showing the amino acid substitutions of Hb S and Hb C.**

Sickle cell syndromes of intermediate severity also had been recognized, and in Neel's study of 33 families, in which both parents of children with sickle cell anemia were examined, in 2 families one parent failed to sickle. The nonsickling parents proved to have hemoglobin C trait and the propositi, sickle cell-hemoglobin C disease. The segregation of these genes in families is seen in Figure 1. In the ensuing years it has been shown that matings of individuals with sickle cell-hemoglobin C disease with normal spouses produce only offspring with sickle cell trait or hemoglobin C trait, thus demonstrating that the genes for Hb S and Hb C are alleles.

The structural studies revealed that the very same amino acid residue altered in Hb S was replaced in the case of Hb C by a lysine residue (Fig. 3). Since the side chain of lysine is electropositive and the glutamic acid electronegative, the glutamic to lysine substitution results in Hb C being twice as electropositive as Hb S, thus accounting for its decreased electrophoretic mobility. These correlations firmly established the principle that mutant genes may cause only small abnormalities in the primary structure of proteins which in turn may lead to major phenotypic abnormalities.

Abnormal Hemoglobin: Associated Polypeptide Substitutions

The hemoglobin molecule is composed of 4 polypeptide chains, 2 alpha and 2 beta, having 141 and 146 amino acid residues, respectively (12). The adult hemoglobin molecule (Hb A) may be designated $\alpha_2{}^A\beta_2{}^A$. A system of nomenclature has been established in which abnormal hemoglobins are designated either alphabetically or by geographical names. The nomenclature also provides for designating the precise substitution when it is known. Thus, Hb S may also be designated as $\alpha_2{}^A\beta_2{}^S$ or as $\alpha_2{}^A\beta_2{}^{6\mathrm{Glu}\to\mathrm{Val}}$, indicating that the substitution has occurred in the sixth residue from the free amino terminal end of the beta chain.

Approximately 150 abnormal hemoglobins have been described (12,23). Of these, approximately one-half are due to amino acid substitutions in the alpha- and one-half in the beta polypeptide chains (Table 1). Two different, and in point of fact, unlinked genetic loci determine the structure of the two types of chains. The data supporting this conclusion comes from studies of critical families in which one spouse has two abnormal hemoglobin genes, one affecting alpha and one affecting beta chains (23). Four types of offspring are produced: heterozygotes for each of the mutant genes, offspring possessing both mutants, and homozygotes for the normal alleles. The latter two types, having both or neither abnormal genes, prove that the two mutants cannot be alleles. The individuals heterozygous at both the alpha and beta loci have a very distinctive electrophoretic pattern with four types of hemoglobin molecules: $\alpha_2{}^A\beta_2{}^A$, $\alpha_2{}^X\beta_2{}^A$, $\alpha_2{}^A\beta_2{}^Y$, and $\alpha_2{}^X\beta_2{}^Y$, where the last is a hybrid molecule composed of both alpha- and beta-chain abnormalities (12). These findings imply that the alpha and beta chains combine at random after synthesis and a protein molecule may be the product of more than one genetic loci. Conversely, a gene may be defined as the amount of genetic information required to code the structure of a polypeptide chain.

Because amino acid substitution altering net ionic charge anywhere in the molecule (Table 1) will alter electrophoretic mobility, assumptions cannot be made from the electrophoretic pattern alone regarding the identity of given abnormalities. For this reason mild sickle cell syndromes with the electrophoretic pattern of sickle cell anemia may be the result of heterozygosity for $\underline{\mathrm{Hb}_\beta}{}^S$ and other $\underline{\mathrm{Hb}_\beta}$ structural mutants with similar net charge. Such is the case in sickle cell-hemoglobin D disease. To diagnose properly such abnormalities, family studies seeking to detect heterozygotes which do not sickle or the use of other techniques which will separate the two hemoglobins, such as acid agar gel electrophoresis or column chromotography, are needed.

FETAL HEMOGLOBIN

In the fetus, another type of hemoglobin predominates, fetal hemoglobin or Hb F. This molecule is composed of two alpha chains and

Table 1. Amino Acid Substitutions of Abnormal Human Hemoglobins

		Amino acid substitution	
Abnormal Hb	Position	HbA →	Abnormal Hb
Alpha chain variants			
J-Toronto	5	Ala	Asp
J-Paris	12	Ala	Asp
J-Oxford	15	Gly	Asp
I	16	Lys	Glu
J-Medellin	22	Gly	Asp
Memphis	23	Glu	Gln
G-Honolulu, G-Hongkong, G-Singapore	30	Glu	Gln
L-Ferrara, Umi, Kokura, Michigan-1, Tagawa II, Yukuhashi II, Beilinson	47	Asp	Gly
Mexico	54	Gln	Glu
Shimonoseki, Hikoshima	54	Gln	Arg
Norfolk, Kagoshima, Nishiki I, II, III	57	Gly	Asp
M-Boston, Leipzig-2, M-Osaka, M-Koln	58	His	Tyr
N-Seattle	61	Lys	Glu
G-Philadelphia, G-Bristol, G-Azuokoli, D-St. Louis, D-Washington	68	Asn	Lys
Ube II	68	Asn	Asp
M-Iwate, M-Kankakee, M-Oldenberg	87	His	Tyr
Chesapeake	92	Arg	Leu
J-Cape Town	92	Arg	Gln
Chiapas	114	Pro	Arg
J-Tongariki	115	Ala	Asp
O-Indonesia	116	Glu	Lys
Beta chain variants			
Tokuchi	2	His	Tyr
S	6	Glu	Val
C	6	Glu	Lys
C-Harlem	6 / 73	Glu / Asp	Val / Asn
G-San Jose	7	Glu	Gly
Siriraj	7	Glu	Lys
Porto Alegre	9	Ser	Cys
N-New Haven, J-Baltimore	16	Gly	Asp
E-Saskatoon	22	Glu	Lys
Freiburg	23	Val	Deletion
E-Nagasaki	26	Glu	Lys

Table 1. (*Continued*)

Abnormal Hb	Position	Amino acid substitution HbA → Abnormal Hb	
Hammersmith	42	Phe	Ser
G-Galveston, G-Port Arthur, G-Texas	43	Glu	Ala
K-Ibadan	46	Gly	Glu
G-Copenhagen	47	Asp	Asn
J-Bangkok	56	Gly	Asp
Hikari, Ube-3	61	Lys	Asn
M-Saskatoon, M-Kurume, M-Chicago, M-Emory, M-Radon, M-Hita, M-Arhus	63	His	Tyr
Zurich	63	His	Arg
M-Milwaukee-1	67	Val	Glu
Sydney	67	Val	Ala
J-Cambridge	69	Gly	Asp
J-Iran	77	His	Asp
G-Accra	79	Asp	Asn
D-Ibadan	87	Thr	Lys
Gunn-Hill	91–95 or 93–97		Deletion
M-Hyde Park	92	His	Tyr
N-Baltimore, N-Memphis	95	Lys	Glu
Köln	98	Val	Met
Yakima	99	Asp	His
D-Punjab, -Cyprus, -Chicago, -Los Angeles, -Portugal, -N. Carolina	121	Glu	Gln
O-Arabia, -Bulgaria, -New York	121	Glu	Lys
K-Woolwich	132	Lys	Gln
Hope	136	Gly	Asp
Kenwood	143	His	Asp
Ranier	145	Tyr	His
Gamma chain variants			
F-Texas	5	Glu	Lys
F-Galveston	6	Glu	Lys
Delta chain variants			
Sphakia	2	His	Arg
B?	16	Gly	Arg
Flatbush	22	Ala	Glu

two still different chains, the gamma chains. It is the latter which confer upon fetal hemoglobin its unusual properties, such as alkali resistance. Very early in gestation there is also a primitive or "embryonic" hemoglobin which contains two alpha chains and two still different chains, referred to as epsilon chains (11). Alpha chains are therefore produced continuously throughout the life of the individual, but the other chains are switched on and off during the process of differentiation. The relative amounts of embryonic hemoglobin has not been well established, but, as can be seen in Figure 4, at about 12 weeks of gestation Hb A appears, which is to say that the beta locus is switched on. At birth Hb A comprises approximately 25% of the total hemoglobin. Fetal hemoglobin synthesis is then phased out more rapidly, and by the age of 12 months, the adult levels of below 2% are approached. Relatively few structural variants of fetal hemoglobin have been described, probably because the small amounts present in adults make detection difficult.

In approximately one-half of the Hb_β^S homozygotes, the amount of Hb F persisting into adult life is increased, the amount present seldom exceeding 10%. Hemoglobin F levels also are increased in heterozygotes for the beta-thalassemia gene and markedly increased in the homozygotes. Approximately 1 in 500 Negroes has a persistent high fetal hemoglobin gene which allows 15–30% of Hb F to remain throughout adult life. This phenotype is accompanied by no other hematologic abnormalities.

FETAL HEMOGLOBIN AND ACQUIRED DISEASE

Fetal hemoglobin production may also be enhanced by acquired disease. Occasionally, patients with acquired hemolytic anemia, aplastic anemia and pernicious anemia may have increased amounts of Hb F. Approximately 10 per cent of pregnant women have slightly elevated levels, occurring too early in pregnancy to be attributed to leakage from the fetal circulation (22). Patients with hydatid moles (4) and trophoblastic tumors (23) also may have elevated levels of Hb F, suggesting that its production is stimulated by a product of the trophoblast.

HEMOGLOBIN A₂

Approximately 3% of the hemoglobin of adults is composed of a minor component, hemoglobin A_2 (Fig. 2). This component migrates with the same velocity as Hb C on electrophoresis at alkaline pH. It is important because heterozygotes for the beta-thalassemia gene, which we shall define below, possess twice the normal amount of

26

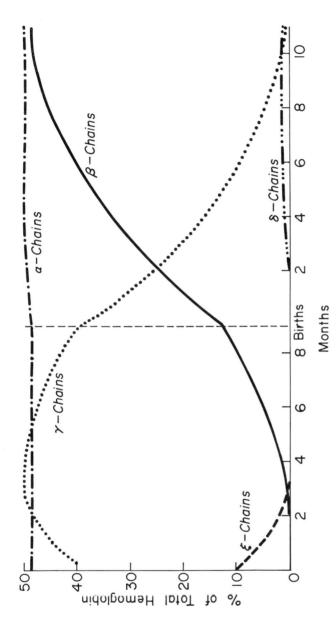

Fig. 4. Changes in distribution of hemoglobin polypeptide chains during pregnancy and in the neonate, showing proportion of total hemoglobin present as each respective chain. Amount of alpha chains present during pregnancy is not quite equal to amount of non-alpha chains until after birth.

this component, that is approximately 5% of their total hemoglobin. Hemoglobin A_2 consists of two alpha chains and two still different chains referred to as delta chains. The amino acid sequence of the delta chains differs from that of the beta chains at only ten residues (12,13). Approximately 2% of Negroes possess a mutant at the Hb_δ locus, referred to as Hb B_2, which migrates still more slowly than $\overline{Hb\ A_2}$. Matings of persons having hemoglobins A, S, A_2 and B_2 produce only offspring with either hemoglobins A, S, and A_2 or hemoglobins A, A_2, and Hb B_2, indicating that the beta and delta structural loci are closely linked (3). No crossovers have been found among some 36 offspring studied to date.

The differences cited between the various types of chains and the linkage relationship of the beta and delta loci have lead to the notion that these have all evolved from a single primitive heme protein by repetitive genetic duplication or translocation (13). The differences now observed are presumably the result of divergence due to the accumulation of mutational changes and the pressures of natural selection.

In summary, the contents of each red cell are determined by five structural loci which are capable of directing the synthesis of varying amounts of subunits, depending upon the stage of development and other stimuli, as yet poorly defined. The subunits recombine at random with some constraints. The distribution of hemoglobin components, therefore, reflects the relative rates of translation of these loci. That these rates are influenced by genetic mechanisms is evidenced by the interactions of thalassemia and the abnormal hemoglobins to which we now turn.

THALASSEMIA SYNDROMES: DISORDERS OF HEMOGLOBIN CONTROL MECHANISMS

Clinical Classification

Thalassemia is a generic term for what is recognized increasingly as a heterogeneous group of hypochromic, microcytic, inherited anemias not due to iron deficiency. Historically, thalassemia has been clinically classified into major, intermediate, and minor forms (Table .2). In *thalassemia major* the total hemoglobin levels are less than 7 grams per 100 ml., the morphologic abnormality is severe, and hepatosplenomegaly is marked. Life can be maintained only with a sustained program of periodic transfusions. *Thalassemia minor* is

Findings	Major	Intermedia	Minor	Minima
Hemoglobin (Gm. %)	< 7	7–10	10–13	12–15
Reticulocytes (%)	2–25	2–15	2–5	< 2
Nucleated RBCs	++++	0 → ++	0	0
RBC morphologic abnormality	++++	++++	++	0
Jaundice	++	0 → +	0	0
Splenomegaly	++++	++	+	0
Skeletal changes	++++	++	Rare	0
Hemoglobin F (%)	50–100	2–50	2–10	1–5

Table 2. Clinical Classification of Thalassemia

characterized by mild hypochromia and microcytosis, inconstant splenomegaly, and hemoglobin levels varying from 10–15 grams per 100 ml. The intermediate form is, as its name implies, between these extremes. Some hematologists prefer to subdivide the minor form into *thalassemia minima*, if anemia is not present.

With greater understanding of the genetic nature of thalassemia, it has become clear that the major form represents the homozygous state and the minor and minima classes are heterozygous phenotypes. The intermediate forms have proven to be mostly combinations of thalassemia and abnormal hemoglobins as well as homozygosity for diverse genes which impart less severe phenotypic effects. With the advent of electrophoretic techniques and better understanding of the nature of thalassemia, a new nosology is still evolving, based upon the genetic and biochemical interactions between hemoglobin structural and regulator loci.

Beta Thalassemia

The relationship of thalassemia to the hemoglobinopathies (12,18,20,28) emerged with the observation of large amounts of fetal hemoglobin in Cooley's anemia or beta-thalassemia homozygotes. Then, the discovery that individuals having only one $HB_\beta{}^S$ gene and one thalassemia gene produced less Hb A than a simple heterozygote for $Hb_\beta{}^S$ lead to the concept of thalassemia as a more or less specific depression of β^A chain synthesis, and thus, the designation beta thalassemia. The term assumed an added dimension with the demonstration that the thalassemia allele is either an allele of the Hb_β structural locus, or is on a closely linked locus. The evidence for this is that matings of sickle-cell-β-thalassemics with normal spouses produce offspring with either sickle cell trait or thalassemia minor; children having both or neither gene, that is genetic crossovers, have not as yet been reported (18,20). An absolute increase in the amount of Hb A_2 in the blood of heterozygotes, from the normal levels of 2–3.5% to approximately 4–6% of the total hemoglobin is one of the most pathognomonic features of beta thalassemia. In only approximately one-half of the cases is the fetal hemoglobin increased, generally to less than 10% of the total hemoglobin. The reasons for the increases in these minor components are not clear. They do not compensate for, nor are they relative to the depression of synthesis of beta chains. More recently the increased amounts of Hb F have been shown to be concentrated in a small population of cells (2). The basis of this mosaicism is not understood as yet.

"Mediterranean" and "African" variants

Studies of families containing homozygotes for beta thalassemia show that, at the very least, there are two types of beta thalassemia. Although the simple heterozygotes are phenotypically identical, the two types are discernable on the basis of phenotype of the homozygote and by variation in the interaction with structural hemoglobinopathies. The "Mediterranean" type of beta thalassemia found in the northern Mediterranean Basin, in Greece, Italy, and Turkey is manifested in the homozygous state as severe thalassemia major or Cooley's anemia. When combined with the gene for sickle cell anemia, this type depresses completely the amount of Hb A produced; but for the increase in the amount of Hb A_2, the electrophoretic pattern might be indistinguishable from that of sickle cell anemia. For this reason we do not refer to an electrophoretic pattern as being of the "SS" type, since this connotes two $\underline{Hb_\beta}^S$ genes which is not the case in sickle cell-thalassemia. Sickle cell-thalassemia rather than sickle cell anemia should be suspected when the clinical manifestations are mild, when splenomegaly is present after the age of 15, or when hypochromia or target cells are excessive in patients with the "all S" electrophoretic pattern. The diagnosis is best verified by demonstrating thalassemia in either parents, siblings, or offspring of the patient.

In the majority of American Negroes with sickle cell-thalassemia, the synthesis of Hb A has not been so severely depressed, so that 15–25% of the total hemoglobin is Hb A. This pattern, with more Hb S than Hb A, is pathognomonic. The amount of Hb A_2 should be twice that usually observed in simple sickle cell trait, which, incidentally, is usually somewhat higher than normal for technical reasons. The homozygote for the "African" type of beta thalassemia is manifested clinically as thalassemia intermedia, with 9–10 grams

30

per 100 ml. of hemoglobin, and moderate splenomegaly (9). The levels of Hb F in either type of sickle cell-thalassemia are somewhat higher than in sickle cell anemia.

Alpha Thalassemia

The converse of beta thalassemia, alpha thalassemia, is defined in chemical rather than genetic terms. Our understanding of alpha thalassemia has evolved from an understanding of hemoglobin H disease, a distinctive type of thalassemia intermedia (Table 2) found in Southeast Asia and in populations with Chinese admixture. It is also present in the Middle East and in the Mediterranean Basin, although less frequently. Upon incubation of these cells with oxidative dyes, as in wet reticulocyte preparations, distinctive inclusions appear in the red cells which have been proven to be precipitates of denatured hemoglobin. The electrophoretic pattern shows small amounts, generally less than 20%, of Hb H which migrates faster than Hb A at alkaline pH (net charge of -4 in Fig. 2). The inclusions are due to the instability of this component.

BART'S HEMOGLOBIN

Younger patients have large amounts of another abnormal component migrating between Hb A and Hb H, Bart's hemoglobin. As the patient matures the amount of Bart's decreases and the Hb H appears and increases. The amount of Hb A_2 is below normal, fetal hemoglobin per se is usually not elevated; the remainder of the hemoglobin is Hb A. Hemoglobin H contains no alpha chains but, rather, is a tetramer structured solely by beta chains (β_4^A). Similarly, Hb Bart's is derived from the gamma locus (γ_4^F). Therefore, Hb H disease appears to be the result of a decrease in the rate of synthesis of alpha polypeptide chains relative to beta and gamma, and thus the concept of alpha thalassemia.

Family studies of patients with Hb H disease show that in the majority of families one parent appears normal and only one parent has overt evidence of thalassemia (20,25). This consists of only mild microcytosis, aniso-poikilocytosis, and slightly decreased levels of Hb A_2. Since these morphologic abnormalities are also found in iron deficiency states, the diagnosis is often not unequivocal. The dissimilarity of parents suggests that either two different genes are responsible for Hb H disease or, that the phenotypic expression for alpha thalassemia is more variable than is the case with beta thalassemia. Support for the former interpretation is obtained by the observation in Southeast Asia of hydrops fetalis, accompanied by hematologic abnormalities of thalassemia and the presence of large amounts of Bart's hemoglobin, of the order of 80% (15,19). These hydropic feti are believed to be homozygotes for the type of alpha thalassemia present in the abnormal parent of the propositi with Hb H disease (15). If this interpretation is correct, the phenotype for the homozygote for the silent gene carried by the normal parent is as yet unknown.

In heterozygous variant

The most specific index of heterozygosity for alpha thalassemia is the presence of increased amounts of Hb Bart's in cord blood–approximately 5–10% (27). Even this is not unequivocal because normally small amounts are present, indicating some inequality in the amount of alpha and non-alpha chains produced during embryogenesis. This sign disappears with advancing age, however, and a pathognomonic abnormality analogous to the increased level of Hb A_2 is lacking in the alpha-thalassemia heterozygote.

In doubly heterozygous variant

The concept of alpha thalassemia rests entirely upon inference from biochemical observations. Genetic evidence that the responsible gene is allelic or closely linked to the $\underline{Hb_\alpha}$ structural locus is as yet lacking. This must await the appearance of families in which one parent has both alpha thalassemia and a $\underline{Hb_\alpha}$ structural mutant. That alpha thalassemia does interact with such structural mutants is evidenced by the presence of greater than 50% of the abnormal hemoglobin in such doubly heterozygous persons, analogous to the interaction of beta thalassemia and $\underline{Hb_\beta}$ structural mutants.

Alpha thalassemia and Hb_β structural mutant combination

Another indication of the presence of the alpha thalassemia gene comes from the combination of alpha thalassemia and Hb_β structural mutants. In Thailand individuals having two alpha thalassemia genes in addition to one $\underline{Hb_\beta}^E$ have the hematologic findings of thalassemia intermedia and produce only about 15% of Hb E, and approximately 10% of Bart's Hb, the remainder being Hb A (20). Simple heterozygotes for $\underline{Hb_\beta}^E$ have minimal morphologic abnormalities but no anemia, and approximately 30–35% of Hb E, whereas heterozygotes for $\underline{Hb_\beta}^E$ and alpha thalassemia genes have only 22–28% of Hb E (20). The limited family data published to date suggests also that two types of alpha thalassemia might exist, one resulting in approximately 28% Hb E and one with about 22%.

A type of alpha thalassemia is also present in the American Negro. Approximately 2% of cord bloods contain significantly elevated amounts of Hb Bart's (27). Additionally, in Negroes with sickle cell trait at least two modes of distribution of the amount of Hb S are present. In simple sickle cell trait, 38–42% of the hemoglobin is Hb S, while in the sickle cell-alpha thalassemia combination, this is decreased to 25% (20,27). Despite the prevalence of this gene in the Negro, Hb H disease has not been described, nor has the Bart's-hydrops fetalis syndrome been detected.

Other variants of thalassemia have been reported having other combinations of hemoglobin aberrations. Various terminologies have been applied to these, but detailed critique is beyond the scope of this review, and the reader is referred to reviews on the subject (12,16,18,20,28). It is important to stress that when hematologic abnormalities are encountered having features of thalassemia but which do not fit the picture of alpha and beta thalassemia as outlined above, the thalassemic nature of the abnormality can be demonstrated by examining appropriate family members. One looks for parent to offspring transmission of whatever abnormalities are present, and frequently the nature of the defect can only be inferred when chance brings it into coexistence with another abnormality, such as a hemoglobin structural variant.

The biochemical nature of thalassemia has not as yet been demonstrated. The evidence indicates that alpha and beta chains are produced at diminished rates (28). At one time the favored hypothesis was that an amino acid substitution in the respective chains not altering net charge but retarding synthesis was responsible. This has been discounted but on rather thin evidence. Now the favored hypothesis is that a base pair substitution in a structural gene codon has resulted in a degenerate code word (26), resulting in the amino acid normally translated at that residue but at a diminished rate of synthesis. Other evidence, on the other hand, is compatible with the possibility that thalassemia is a derangement of the operator-regulator mechanism governing protein synthesis. The solution of this problem remains an exciting challenge yet to be realized.

POPULATION GENETICS

To assess fully the public health aspects of inherited diseases it is necessary to understand the principles of population genetics, which in essence is the study of the genetic composition of groups of people and of the factors which cause changes in this genetic composition. Knowledge of the frequency of various genes in a population allows anticipation of the prevalence of various genotypes. Also, careful analysis of genetic data may allow definition of the forces tending to alter gene frequency such as selection, mutation, genetic drift, and population migration.

Gene Pool and Genotype Distribution

Crucial to population genetics is the notion of a gene pool. This envisions a population of individuals as contributors to a pool of genes, such that each person contributes two alleles at *each* locus. Each new generation represents a random sample, taken two at a time, from the pool of the previous generation. The Hardy-Weinberg Law, described independently in 1908 by Hardy and Weinberg, states that under certain conditions the frequency of genes in the population is invariant from one generation to the next, and that the various genotypes are distributed according to a polynomial distribution, depending upon the relative frequency of alleles in the gene pool. Thus, if there are only 2 alleles at a given locus (A and a), and if p is the proportion of A alleles in the pool and q the proportion of a alleles (where $p + q = 1$), the frequency of the three possible genotypes—AA, Aa, and aa—is p^2, $2pq$, and q^2, respectively. These, it will be noted, are the terms of the binomial expansion: $(p + q)^2 = p^2 + 2pq + q^2 = 1$. For 3 alleles the algebra is only slightly more complicated. For hemoglobins A, S, and C the distribution would be as follows: $p^2(AA) + 2pq(AS) + q^2(SS) + 2pr(AC) + 2qr(SC) + r^2(CC) = 1$. In practice the gene frequency is estimated by enumerating the number of A, S, and C genes in the sample, considering that each normal person possesses 2 $\underline{Hb_\beta}^A$ alleles, each sickle cell trait one $\underline{Hb_\beta}^A$ and one $\underline{Hb_\beta}^S$, etc., and then applying this estimate of p, q, and r to the above equation. In a small sample, only the commonest genotypes may be represented and the rare ones neglected.

SICKLE CELL ANEMIA IN AMERICAN NEGROES

In the American Negro the frequency of sickle cell trait varies considerably, from 6 per cent in Washington, D. C. (17) to 16 per cent in the Gullah Negro of Charleston, S. C. The mean value is approximately 10 per cent, and the mean frequency of Hb C trait is approximately 2 per cent. The estimated gene frequency is one-half the observed trait frequency in a given population because each

34

heterozygote contributes only one abnormal gene to the pool. Therefore, the expected frequency of sickle cell anemia in the American Negro is $(0.05)^2$ or 1 in 400. These calculations are extended in a similar fashion to include the remaining genotypes of the $\underline{Hb_\beta}$ locus and the results detailed in Table 3. The calculation for sickle cell-

Table 3. Anticipated Frequencies of Various Hemoglobin Genotypes in the American Negro

Hemoglobin genotype	S/A	C/A	β-thal. trait	S/S	S/C	S/β-thal.	C/C
Anticipated frequency	$\frac{1}{10}$	$\frac{1}{50}$	$\frac{1}{125}$	$\frac{1}{400}$	$\frac{1}{1000}$	$\frac{1}{2500}$	$\frac{1}{10,000}$

thalassemia is based on the frequency of beta thalassemia minor of 0.8 per cent, found in a random sample of Negroes in St. Louis. This distribution shows that if we sample a population of Negroes, say, through an obstetrics clinic, and if the sample is representative of the population at birth, there should be 2.5 women with sickle cell anemia for each case of sickle cell-hemoglobin C disease. This ratio applies, of course, only if the frequency of sickle cell trait and Hb C-trait are 10 and 2 per cent, respectively.

Studies in United States

With these figures in mind, let us look at the studies which have been done to date. In the United States only two studies are large enough to allow meaningful analysis. McCurdy (17) electrophoresed the blood of 3,333 consecutive admissions to the Prenatal Clinic of the District of Columbia General Hospital. Only 6.4 per cent of these had sickle hemoglobin, suggesting that the degree of Caucasian admixture of the Negro is somewhat higher there than elsewhere in the country. Of the 3,333 admissions, approximately $3,333 \times (.03)^2$ or 3 cases of homozygous sickle cell anemia were anticipated, which is precisely what he found. Overlooking the question of statistical significance, this suggests that all of the Negro females with sickle cell anemia survived to reach the prenatal clinic, a suggestion which is difficult to accept. These results can probably be attributed to biasing of the D. C. General Hospital population by patients with sickle cell anemia referred by the private practitioners or other hospitals in the area. In this series the expected number of sickle cell-hemoglobin C disease was 2 cases; 3 were seen.

35

In the study of Laros, performed at Temple University Hospital in Philadelphia, 3,701 consecutive prenatal patients were screened with sickle cell preparations and 9 per cent were found to be positive. Therefore, 7.4 patients with sickle cell anemia were expected; 3 were observed. This difference is not statistically significant. Similarly, 7 cases of sickle cell-hemoglobin C disease were observed; only 3.3 were expected. This excess is significant at the 1 per cent level of probability (chi square = 5.3; d.f. = 1), suggesting that in this series also, ascertainment bias was present. If this is so, the previous observation—that only one-half of the patients homozygous for the $Hb_\beta{}^S$ gene survived to adulthood—also can be expected to be inflated by the same bias, whatever the source.

The above considerations cannot be considered definitive, but rather, emphasize the state of ignorance in which we find ourselves in attempting to determine the realities of life when viewed from the perspective of a hospital population. Population genetics must be taken into account both in evaluation of published data and in experimental design. We shall return to further considerations pertinent to population genetics in the next section.

INFLUENCE OF HEMOGLOBINOPATHIES ON REPRODUCTION

To counsel properly a prospective mother afflicted with a chronic hereditary disorder, the physician must consider both the genetic risk to future offspring, and the interaction between the disease and the proffered pregnancy. Specifically we are interested in the influence of the hemoglobinopathies on fertility, abortion, maternal morbidity, maternal mortality, and perinatal mortality.

Table 4 summarizes the current concept of both the clinical severity of various hemoglobinopathies in the nonpregnant state, and their influences on reproduction (5,6,10,14,17,24,29). We hasten to point out that there is really very little objective data on which to base conclusions regarding the maternal and fetal effects on the abnormal hemoglobin syndromes. Much of the literature dealing with pregnancy and hemoglobinopathies consists of case reports and empirical observations. This mode of collection introduces an obvious bias in ascertainment which tends to overemphasize complications and yields little information about fertility, abortion rates, and perinatal mortality.

There is general agreement that the maternal mortality rate is increased when pregnancy is associated with sickle cell anemia and S/C disease as compared to both nonpregnant women with the same hemoglobinopathies and to normal parturients. Unfortunately, the mag-

36

Table 4. Influence of Hemoglobinopathies on Reproduction

Hemoglobin pattern	Fertility	Abortion rate	Maternal morbidity*	Maternal mortality	Perinatal mortality	Clinical severity, nonpregnant
S/S	decreased	increased	increased A, M, S, C, P, Ph, Pn	10–20%	20–30%	+++
A/S	normal	unchanged	slight increase Pn	unchanged	unchanged	±
S/Thal.	normal	unknown	increased probably like S/C	unknown	unknown	+ to ++
S/C	normal	unchanged	increased A, M, S, C, P, Pn, Hp	2–10%	slight increase	± to ++
C/C	normal	unknown	slight increase A, M	unchanged	unchanged	+
Thal. minor	normal	unchanged	slight increase A	unchanged	unchanged	− to +
E/E	unknown	unknown	slight increase A, M	unknown	unknown	+
E/Thal.	unknown	unknown	increased A, M	unknown	unknown	+ to +++

*A–anemia; M–megaloblastic crisis; S–acute sequestration; C–bone, abdominal, and cerebral crises; P–pneumonia; Ph–antepartum hemorrhage; Pn–pyelonephritis; Hp–postpartum hemorrhage.

nitude of the risk is not known, nor is the fertility of these women known. With the advent of a more liberal attitude towards therapeutic abortion and the availability of effective methods of contraception, this information is needed in order to counsel such patients properly.

Sickle Cell Trait

The effect of sickle cell trait upon fertility is somewhat easier to evaluate for several reasons. The trait is much more common than sickle cell anemia and the other hemoglobinopathies, and the trait in itself produces minimal morbidity, thus making ascertainment bias less likely. A considerable amount of information has accumulated from Africa which, in brief, indicates that sickle cell trait confers approximately a 15 per cent greater longevity and that heterozygous women appear to have fertilities approximately 13 per cent greater than normal women (1,23). The interaction of sickle trait with malaria precludes extrapolation of these data to the Negro population of the United States and the reader is referred to reviews of the subject by Rucknagel and Neel (23), Allison (1), and Livingstone (16) for more detailed discussion.

The largest study of women with sickle cell trait in the U. S. is that of McCurdy (17). In his study, 206 women with sickle cell trait had 4.11 pregnancies per person, compared with 3.98 for the normal homozygotes. This difference, not statistically significant, may be attributable to a 0.5 year difference in mean age of the mothers. The total fetal loss was not significantly different. Forty-three mothers with Hb C trait had 4.98 pregnancies per mother and a significantly increased number of premature infants. In this study the frequency of Hb C trait was significantly higher in the obstetrical group than in a control group of hospital employees. In addition, the obstetrical patients with Hb C trait had more anemia, and were 2 years older than the obstetrical group homozygous for $Hb_\beta{}^A$. Again, sample bias seems to be present, although difficult to define. One possible source might be that there are 2 populations of Negroes in Washington, one of which has less Caucasian ancestry and therefore more Hb C trait, and also less favorable economic circumstances correlating with more anemia and more premature infants. In his study, women with sickle cell anemia had only 2.74 children per person and significantly more fetal wastage and complications of pregnancy. This group is not comparable to the other obstetrical patients with which it was controlled inasmuch as only 3 of the 19 women with sickle cell anemia were ascertained through the obstetrical service, the remainder com-

Table 5. Pregnancy Wastage Classified According to Mating Type of a Triracial Isolate*

Number of matings, pregnancies, and fetal wastage	$AA \times AA$	$AA\,\sigma \times AS\,\male$	$AS\,\sigma \times AA\,\male$	$AS \times AS$	χ^2; d.f.†
Matings	103	37	27	10	
Total pregnancies	714	251	210	83	
Mean no. pregnancies	6.92	6.79	7.78	8.30	
Miscarriages	52	19	18	3	2.20; 3
No. miscarriages per pregnancy	0.073	0.076	0.086	0.0362	
Stillbirths	22	5	9	8	11.71; 3‡
No. stillbirths per pregnancy	0.039	0.020	0.043	0.097	
Neonatal deaths	14	4	2	2	0.23; 3
No. neonatal deaths per pregnancy	0.0196	0.016	0.009	0.023	
Total fetal wastage	88	28	29	13	1.51; 3
Total fetal wastage per pregnancy	0.123	0.112	0.138	0.157	

* From Rucknagel (21).
† Chi squares calculated by 2 × 4 comparison of the number of fetal deaths with the remaining pregnancies in each mating type.
‡ $0.01 > P > 0.001$.

ing from the hematology service records. Had McCurdy not so enriched his sample, on the other hand, he would not have had a sufficient number of observations.

In assessing differential fertility, greater precision can be obtained by taking the genotype of the father into account, especially when the odds are high that he will also be a heterozygote. The value of analyzing the data in such a fashion is shown in Table 5, in which the fetal wastage and fertility data are summarized from a study of a triracial isolate in Southern Maryland having an inordinately high frequency of the sickle cell gene (21). Although a number of trends are observed, only the number of stillbirths when both parents have the trait is significantly increased. This finding suggests that the protection believed to be offered the homozygote for the $\underline{Hb_\beta}^s$ gene by the fetal hemoglobin present is not absolute. This also emphasizes another point, namely, the contribution of the genotype of the child to fertility.

The above considerations underline the importance of experimental design in undertaking studies of such complex phenomena.

GENETIC COUNSELLING

The obstetrician-gynecologist is in an ideal position to provide genetic counselling, and is frequently requested to do so by his patients. Such a request may be motivated by either the delivery of an infant with a genetic abnormality, or a couple's suspicion or knowledge that they may be carriers of a genetic disorder.

Prospective parents seeking genetic counselling are asking in essence three questions: (1) what is the *chance* that a child of this mating will be afflicted by the abnormality in question? (2) what is the anticipated course of the disease in the affected parent, and specifically, what is the influence of pregnancy on the disease's course? and (3) what is the influence of the disease on the prospective pregnancy?

Having been given the answers to the above questions, the couple will then frequently ask the physician or geneticist what their future reproductive course should be. We firmly believe that a couple should be apprised of *all* available facts bearing on the issue, but, with rare exception, the counsellor *should not* attempt to pass judgment as to the advisability of parenthood. This decision normally belongs to the individual couple.

The hemoglobinopathies lend themselves especially well to genetic counselling. The mode of inheritance is well documented, and it is usually simple to identify the heterozygous state. Applying the principles of Mendelian genetics to the more common mating types involving hemoglobins S, C, and thalassemia, Table 6 shows the *a priori* risk of having affected children. It should be emphasized that the risk for each successive child is independent of the outcome of previous pregnancies.

Table 6. Expected Phenotype Ratios Among Offspring of Matings of More Common Hemoglobin Phenotypes

Mating type \ Zygote phenotype	A/A	A/S	S/S	A/C	S/C	S–β–thal.	β–thal. minor	C/C	C/β–thal.
A/A × A/S	½	½							
A/S × A/S	¼	½	¼						
S/S × A/A		1							
S/S × A/S		½	½						
S/S × S/S			1						
A/S × A/C	¼	¼		¼	¼				
S/C × A/A		½		½					
S/C × A/S		¼	¼	¼	¼				
S/C × A/C		¼		¼	¼			¼	
S/β–thal. × A/A		½					½		
S/β–thal. × A/S		¼	¼			¼	¼		
S/β–thal. × S/S			½			½			
S/β–thal. × S/C			¼		¼	¼			¼

The following hypothetical case history demonstrates some of the principals involved.

CASE HISTORY (HYPOTHETICAL)

A 22-year-old Negro female presented herself for evaluation prior to undertaking her first pregnancy. She is asymptomatic and gives no past history or family history of anemia. Her husband had a sister who died at age 9 with sickle cell anemia.

The general physical and pelvic examinations were entirely normal.

Routine urinalysis, hemoglobin, hematocrit, white cell count, serology, cervical cytology, and tuberculin test are all normal or negative. The sickle cell preparation is positive. Because of the positive sickle cell preparation, an electrophoresis is obtained which shows the patient to have S/C disease.

A hemoglobin electrophoresis of her husband's blood shows him to have sickle cell trait.

Specific Information to Couple

The following information is made available to the couple: (1) The anticipated clinical courses of both sickle cell trait and S/C disease were explained in detail; (2) Referring to Table 6 we found the expected ratio of hemoglobin patterns in their offspring would be: ¼ S/S: ¼ S/C: ¼ A/S: ¼ A/C; (3) The clinical significance of sickle cell anemia and of hemoglobin C trait were explained; (4) The evidence concerning the adverse influence of pregnancy on the course of S/C disease was presented; (5) They were advised that S/C disease appears to have no effect on abortion rates, and only slightly increases the prematurity and perinatal mortality rates; and (6) The future use of oral contraceptives was proscribed because of the growing body of evidence implicating their use with thrombo-embolic disease. A definite cause-effect relationship between oral contraceptives, sickle cell hemoglobinopathies, and thrombosis is unproven, and there have been only a few case reports of thrombosis in women with sickle cell variants on oral contraceptives (8).

Certainly, the above hypothetical case represents an unusual mating and the family history makes consideration of the hemoglobinopathies imperative. In the much more likely mating of 2 individuals with sickle cell trait, there is also a 1 in 4 probability of having an offspring with sickle cell anemia. At the very least, a sickle cell preparation should be part of the routine laboratory studies on all new Negro obstetric and gynecologic patients, for only in this way will the asymptomatic heterozygote be detected and properly counselled.

SUMMARY AND HORIZONS

We have attempted to detail basic genetic material with special emphasis on the characteristics of structural genes and thalassemia as examples of defective regulatory genes. The foregoing discussion suggests a number of areas where deficiencies of information exist.

To assist in genetic counselling, and to evaluate the magnitude of the public health problem, more data on the size of the risk to both mother and child are desirable. Tabulating published case reports does not provide an adequate estimate because of the biases inherent in such data, and because of the different frequencies based upon the population genetic considerations described above. At the very least, interpretation of the relative incidence of complications should take into account the fact that the various specific syndromes are present in the population in different frequencies. Prospective data based upon randomly or consecutively ascertained parturient women from the population at large rather than a single hospital are desirable.

Barring the development of specific therapy of the sickling disorders, better estimates of the morbidity and mortality rates associated with pregnancy are desirable in order to evaluate the aggressiveness with which the supportive means at hand are utilized. We need to know whether anticoagulation during pregnancy in patients with sickle cell-hemoglobin C disease is beneficial or not. We need to evaluate systematically the use of prophylactic transfusion programs. Such data will accumulate slowly because of the relative rareness of these entities. Perhaps collaborative efforts toward these ends are in order. The impact of these genes upon fertility are questions of considerable importance to the population geneticist.

As noted in the discussion of alpha thalassemia, the frequency of alpha thalassemia is such in the American Negro that one in 10,000 births are expected to be homozygous for this gene. If here, as in Southeast Asia, this genotype is manifested as hydrops fetalis with Bart's hemoglobin (15,19), it is possible that these are being overlooked. We suggest, therefore, that all hydropic Negro fetuses be studied by hemoglobin electrophoresis, especially those who are Coombs test negative or where isoimmunization of the mother is not demonstrable.

Although the "molecular" nature of these genetic aberrations is unfolding rapidly, we still know little about the pathophysiology of the clinical disorders produced. Hopefully, in the near future we will have both a better understanding of the pathophysiology of the hemoglobinopathies and of the influence of pregnancy on these processes.

REFERENCES

1. ALLISON, A. C. Polymorphism and natural selection in human populations. *Cold Spr. Harb. Symp. quant. Biol.* 29:137, 1964.
2. BETKE, K., and KLEIHAUER, E. Fetaler und bleibender Blutfarbstoff in erythrozyten und erythroblasten von menschlichen feten und neugeborenen. *Blut* 4:241, 1958.
3. BOYER, S. H., RUCKANGEL, D. L., WEATHERALL, D. J., and WATSON-WILLIAMS, E. J. Further evidence for linkage between the β and δ loci governing human hemoglobin and the population dynamics of linked genes. *Amer. J. hum. Genet.* 15:438, 1963.

4. BROMBERG, Y. M., YEHUDA, M., SALZBERGER, M., and ABRAHAMOV, A. Alkali resistant type of hemoglobin in women with molar pregnancy. *Blood* 12:1122, 1957.

5. CURTIS, E. M. Pregnancy in sickle cell-hemoglobin C disease. *Amer. J. Obstet. Gynec.* 77:1312, 1959.

6. FULLERTON, W. T., and WATSON-WILLIAMS, E. J. Hemoglobin SC disease and megaloblastic anemia of pregnancy. *J. Obstet. Gynaec. Brit. Emp.* 69:729, 1962.

7. HARRIS, J. W. Role of physical and chemical factors in the sickling phenomenon. *Progr. Hemat.* 2:47, 1959.

8. HAYNES, R. L., and DUNN, J. M. Oral contraceptives, thrombosis, and sickle cell hemoglobinopathies. *J. Amer. med. Ass.* 200:994, 1967.

9. HELLER, P., YAKULIS, V. J., ROSENZWEIG, A. I., ABILDGAARD, C. F., and RUCKNAGEL, D. L. Mild homozygous beta-thalassemia. Further evidence for the heterogeneity of beta-thalassemia genes. *Ann. intern. Med.* 64:52, 1966.

10. HENDRICKSE, J. R., and WATSON-WILLIAMS, E. J. Influence of hemoglobinopathies on reproduction. *Amer. J. Obstet. Gynec.* 94:739, 1966.

11. HUEHNS, E. R., DANCE, N., BEAVEN, G. H., HECHT, F., and MOTULSKY, A. G. Human embryonic hemoglobins. *Cold Spr. Harb. Symp. quant. Biol.* 29:327, 1964.

12. HUEHNS, E. R., and SHOOTER, E. M. Human haemoglobins. *J. Med. Genet.* 2:48, 1965.

13. INGRAM, V. M. *The Hemoglobins in Genetics and Evolution.* Columbia, New York, 1963.

14. LAROS, R. K. Sickle cell-hemoglobin C disease and pregnancy. *Penn. Med.* 70:73, 1967.

15. LIE-INJO, L. E., LIE HONG GIE, AGER, J. A., and LEHMANN, H. α-thalassemia as a cause of hydrops foetalis. *Brit. J. Haemat.* 8:1, 1962.

16. LIVINGSTONE, F. B. *Abnormal Hemoglobins in Human Populations.* Aldine Co., Chicago, 1967, pp. 470.

17. McCURDY, P. R. Abnormal hemoglobins and pregnancy. *Amer. J. Obstet. Gynec.* 90:891, 1964.

18. MOTULSKY, A. G. Current concepts of the genetics of the thalassemias. *Cold Spr. Harb. Symp. quant. Biol.* 29:399, 1964.

19. POOTRAKUL, S., WASI, P., and NA-NAKORN, S. Hemoglobin Bart's hydrops foetalis in Thailand. *Ann. hum. Genet.* 30:293, 1967.

20. RUCKNAGEL, D. L. Current concepts of the genetics of thalassemia. *Ann. N. Y. Acad. Sci.* 119(2):436, 1964.

21. RUCKNAGEL, D. L. Gene for sickle cell hemoglobin in the Wesorts: An extreme example of genetic drift and the founder effect. Ph.D. Thesis, University of Michigan. Dissertation Abstr. 28:500B, 1967.

22. RUCKNAGEL, D. L., and CHERNOFF, A. I. Immunologic studies of hemoglobins. III. Fetal hemoglobin changes in the circulation of pregnant women. *Blood* 10:1092, 1955.

44

23. RUCKNAGEL, D. L., and NEEL, J. V.   Hemoglobinopathies. *Progr. Med. Genet. 1:*158, 1961.
24. SMITH, E. W., and CONLEY, C. I.   Clinical features of genetic variants of sickle cell disease. *Bull. Johns Hopk. Hosp. 94:*289, 1954.
25. WASI, P., NA-NAKORN, S., and SUINGDAMRONG, A.   Thalassemia-hemoglobin H in Thailand: A genetical study. *Nature 204:*907, 1964.
26. WATSON, J. D. *Molecular Biology of the Gene.* W. A. Benjamin, Inc., New York, 1965, pp. 494.
27. WEATHERALL, D. J.   Abnormal haemoglobins in the neonatal period and their relationships to thalassemia. *Brit. J. Haemat. 9:*265, 1963.
28. WEATHERALL, D. J.   Thalassemias. *Progr. Med. Genet. 5:*8, 1967.
29. WHALLEY, P. J., PRITCHARD, J. A., and RICHARDS, J. R.   Sickle cell trait and pregnancy. *J. Amer. med. Ass. 186:*1132, 1963

45

Is Marriage Counseling Feasible in Africa to Prevent Sickle-Cell Disease?

R. E. BROWN, M.D., D.T.M.&H., M.P.H.,
P. J. S. HAMILTON, M.D., Ch.B., D.T.M.&H.,
J. KAGWA, M.D., M. A. WARLEY, M.D., B.A., D.C.H.

SICKLE–CELL disease is a chronic, debilitating hemolytic disease which affects all of the organ systems of the body.[11] There is no known cure. The physician can only provide supportive, prophylactic and symptomatic therapy to attempt to ameliorate the disturbing symptoms and enhance the prognosis for survival.[8, 17]

Although this disease is characterized by periods of remission and exacerbation, during the clinical course the patient has episodes of stasis, local anoxia, hemolysis, anemia, or thrombosis attributed to intravascular sickling phenomena. In general, the prognosis is not favorable, and in Africa a particularly high mortality in early childhood has been reported.[6, 7, 13-16]

Hemoglobin electrophoresis ascertains the presence of normal or abnormal hemoglobins and makes the diagnosis of homozygous sickle-cell disease relatively simple. It is estimated that more than 20 per cent of individuals living in a large belt across tropical Africa have the sickle-cell gene.[2, 4, 5]

Disease prevention is still in its infancy. Although most people accept that prevention is better and far less costly than cure, no country has so far believed enough in this to be guided by preventive principles.[3]

In a disease like sickle-cell anemia which can be detected easily and for which there is no known cure, a program of prevention could help save many lives, relieve much suffering and decrease the burden on the limited medical resources of developing countries in Africa.

Present Study

Genetic selection can help avoid an incurable disease in which it is possible to determine who is carrying the abnormal gene. It follows, therefore, that favorable arguments can be proposed for marriage counseling. With marriage partner selection, it would be possible to discourage marriage between two sickle-cell carriers. To explore how feasible such a program might be in Africa, a preliminary questionnaire was used as an approach.

Individuals in a university having a higher educational background and a degree of sophistication, were assumed to be more likely to appreciate the problem and understand the role which marriage counseling might play. This communication gives the results of a survey conducted among medical, nursing, midwifery and general university students at Makerere University College, Kampala, Uganda.

Each group of students was given separately an introductory didactic lecture in which basic principles of genetics were explained, and sickle-cell disease was described with the aid of clinical color slides. The manner of inheritance, clinical picture, methods of testing the blood, and the absence of curative therapy were all emphasized. Immediately following the lecture, a session of questions and answers was conducted by the four authors. Each question from the audience was answered carefully, with the basic points reiterated several times. After there were no further questions, the questionnaires were distributed. The completed questionnaires were collected immediately afterwards.

→ The second-year medical students had a distinct advantage, as they were taking an introductory course in medical genetics. Most of the nursing and midwifery students had worked on the medical and pediatric wards in Mulago Hospital and had the opportunity to see and care for patients with sickle-cell disease. In general, the university students were meeting this problem for the first time, having neither theoretical background nor practical contact with sickle-cell disease.

Results

A total of 139 questionnaires were completed. The average age of medical students was 23.3 years, of nursing students, 21.3 years, and of general students, 24.5 years. The nurses and midwives were all women, whereas five of the medical and two of the general students were women. The only married student was one of the nurses.

Represented among the three groups were individuals from 32 tribes, and also 22 non-African students.

Question 1. Is there anyone in your family with sickle-cell disease?

There was no significant difference among the three groups. Approximately 5 per cent knew of relatives with the disorder.

Question 2. Do you have any friends with

this disease?

Between 15 and 19 per cent of the medical and nursing students knew persons with the disease. None of the general students were aware of affected friends or relatives.

Question 3. Have you ever had your blood tested for having or carrying this disease?

None of the general students had been tested. Less than 10 per cent of medical and nursing students had had this test.

Question 4. If yes, what was the reason for having this test?

One reason given was that it had been a classroom exercise in pathology. Several stated it was a "matter of interest" or "of curiosity" and one had a "girl friend who was a carrier for sickling." One reply was that it was done "to detect sickle-cell trait."

Question 5. If not tested, would you want to have this done before marriage?

Eighty-five per cent of those answering the question expressed interest in having a blood test for sickling before marriage, including all of the nurses. Sixteen medical students (12.6 per cent) answered that they would not have a test performed, and two were uncertain.

Question 6. If your results were positive for carrying the disease, would you be especially concerned in selecting a marriage partner who had negative results?

An over-all average of 80 per cent replied that they would be concerned in selection of a partner under the stated conditions, and 12 per cent answered that they would not be concerned. All of the general students replied affirmatively.

Question 7. If your results and your future partner's results were positive, would this al-

ter possible plans?

Seventy per cent replied that plans would be affected by such results. Seventeen per cent determined to go ahead in spite of this knowledge; 12 per cent were not certain what they would do under such circumstances. Little difference was found between one group and another in the answers of Questions 6 and 7.

Several students who answered that they did not know what they would do quite reasonably added on their questionnaires: "love would have to be considered," or that "there were many factors involved." Several nurses commented that "this may mean a decision not to have any children."

Question 8. What is meant by the carrier state for sickle-cell factor?

Approximately 75 per cent of all students replied correctly in definition of the carrier state (73.9 per cent), the medical students doing somewhat better than the others. Between one-quarter and one-third of these answering either gave an incorrect answer or admitted not knowing how to define the carrier state.

(This question served also as an evaluation of instruction, to determine whether the individual had understood what had been explained in the lecture and question periods.)

Question 9. Do you know how sickle-cell disease can be prevented?

Question 10. If yes, how can it be prevented?

Slightly less than 70 per cent of the students knew how to prevent sickle-cell disease. Of the nurses, only half knew how to prevent the disease, whereas over 90 per cent of the general students understood this point, and the medical students were between the other groups, close to the mean. The final question was answered in a variety of ways, some carefully outlining the application of premarital blood testing and selective marriage counseling, and other answers confirmed a lack of understanding.

Comments

Linus Pauling has suggested that the use in the U. S. A. of the easy and convenient blood identification for sickle-cell anemia, combined with other premarital checks, could be used as a means of eradicating sickle-cell disease.[10] A similar sugestion was outlined in a recent symposium on hemoglobinopathies by Sinsicalco, who discussed the following approaches to preventing homozygous SS disease:

1. Prevent marriage of heterozygotes;

2. Prevent offspring of any marriage of sickle-cell carriers;

3. Prevent all sickle-cell carriers from having offspring.[12]

Allison, at the same symposium, was of the opinion that the three measures presented above would represent an infringement on individual liberty.[1]

Among these three groups of university students in Kampala, although their backgrounds and knowledge were dissimilar, a distinct similarity was found in the answers to the questions. The large majority of persons were interested in having their blood tested for sickle-cell disease, and between 70 and 80 per cent thought that they would be influenced if their blood tests were positive. Nearly 70 per cent of the students understood how marriage counseling could play a role in this problem.

No conclusions can be reached on the results of the small sample described in the present study. There was an indication that marriage counseling *might* be considered in dealing with sickle-cell disease. At least, this possibility exists among the more educated group of Ugandans.

Another element in the sickle-cell problem

deserves mention. In the theory of "balanced polymorphism," Motulsky considered that the interaction between malaria and sickling trait is such that the frequency of the gene might decrease simply by removing malaria from the environment.[9] Were malaria eradicated in a community the advantage of the sickling heterozygote would be removed and sickling would decrease without manipulation of the mating behavior of the gene carriers in the population.

Conclusion

When dealing with an incurable disease such as sickle-cell anemia, all possible avenues deserve exploration. The possibility exists that a general blood-testing program could be carried out in a premarital group, such as school children, supplemented by counseling services. Were marriage counseling accepted by the upper and educated classes, it is not unlikely that with time this might serve as an inducement for others in the community, eventually influencing the incidence of the disease in the population.

References

1. Allison, A. C.: *In* Abnormal Haemoglobins in Africa, ed. by Jonxis, J. H. P. Oxford, Blackwell, 1965, p. 456.
2. ——: *In* Human Biology, ed. by Harrison, G. A., Weiner, J. S., Tanner, J. M. and Barnicot, N. A. London, Clarendon Press, 1964, p. 240.
3. Bothwell, P. W.: A New Look at Preventive Medicine, London, Pitman Medical Publishers Ltd., 1965.
4. Editorial: Haemoglobin and evolution. Brit. Med. J. 2: 660, 1965.
5. Edington, R. S.: The pathology of sickle cell disease in West Africa. Trans. Roy. Soc. Trop. Med. Hyg. 49: 253, 1955.
6. Jacob, G. F.: A study of the survival rate of cases of sickle-cell anemia. Brit. Med. J. 1: 738, 1957.
7. Jelliffe, D. B.: Sickle-cell disease. Trans. Roy. Soc. Trop. Med. Hyg. 46: 169, 1952.
8. Kagwa, J., Ferguson, A. D., Scott, R. B. and Bullock, W. H.: Studies in sickle cell anemia XXVIII. Clinical observations on prognosis and

outlook beyond childhood. Med. Ann. Dist. Col.

9. Motulsky, A. C.: *In* Abnormal Haemoglobins in Africa, ed. by Jonxis, J. H. P. Oxford, Blackwell, 1965, p. 457.
10. Pauling, L.: End of sickle cell anemia seen by national use of blood test. Med. Trib. 4: 8, 1963. As quoted in The Pediatric Patient, ed. by Gustafson, S. R. and Coursin, D. B. New Jersey, Hoffmann-La-Roche, Inc., 1963.
11. Scott, R. B. and Ferguson, A. D.: Studies in sickle cell anaemia XV. Diagnosis and management of sickle cell anemia in childhood. Quart. Rev. Pediat. 15: 176, 1960.
12. Sinsicalco, M.: *In* Abnormal Haemoglobins in Africa. *Op. cit.* 451.
13. Smith, E. W. and Torbert, J. V.: Study of two abnormal haemoglobins with evidence for a new genetic locus for haemoglobin formation. Bull. Johns Hopkins Hosp. 102: 38, 1958.
14. Thurman, W. C. and Platou, R. V.: Sickle cell disease in the young. Proc. of Hematology (Third Session) Ninth International Congress of Pediat., Montreal, Canada, July, 1959.
15. Tomlinson, W. J.: Abdominal crises in uncomplicated sickle cell anemia. Amer. J. Med. Sci. 209: 722, 1945.
16. Trowell, H. C., Raper, A. B. and Welbourn, H. F.: The natural history of homozygous sickle cell anemia in central Africa. Quart. J. Med. 26: 401, 1957.
17. Warley, M. A., Hamilton, P. J. S., Marsden, P. D., Brown, R. E., Merselis, J. G. and Wilks, N.: Chemoprophylaxis of homozygous sicklers with antimalarials and long-acting penicillin. Brit. Med. J. 2: 86, 1965.

Genetic Counseling and Cancer:

Implications for Cancer Control

HENRY T. LYNCH, M.D., and ANNE J. KRUSH, M.S.

CLINICAL GENETICS has made astounding progress in medicine since the end of World War II. Genetic research has been responsible for fundamental contributions at the basic medical science level. It has served ably as an invaluable tool for the diagnostician, epidemiologist and therapist at the clinical level.[1] The potential for application of clinical genetics is being realized repeatedly at the basic level of family practice.

In spite of this accelerated progress of medical genetics, its application to clinical oncology has progressed more slowly. This is interesting because scientific awareness of the importance of hereditary factors in cancer has existed since the 18th century.[2]

Early investigations in cancer genetics were restricted almost exclusively to studies of animals. The earliest studies of cancer genetics in humans were concerned primarily with site specific malignant neoplasms, such as cancer of the breast, colon, stomach and skin. The value of these initial studies was questionable because of the lack of pathologic documenta-

54

TABLE 1

Autosomal Dominant Disorders	
Familial polyposis coli	Peutz-Jeghers syndrome
Gardner's syndrome	Tylosis (keratosis et palmaris plantaris) and esophageal cancer
Hereditary exostosis	
Nevoid basal cell carcinoma syndrome	Von-Recklinghausen's neurofibromatosis
Hereditary polyendocrine adenomatosis	Retinoblastoma
Medullary thyroid carcinoma with amyloid production and pheochromocytoma	Carotid body tumors
	Lindau von Hippel disease
	Tuberous sclerosis

Autosomal Recessive Disorders	
Xeroderma pigmentosum	Chediak-Higashi syndrome
Bloom's syndrome	Wiskott-Aldrich syndrome
Fanconi's aplastic anemia	Ataxia telangiectasia (Louis-Bar syndrome)

Sex-linked Disorders
Agammaglobulinemia (Bruton's type)

A listing of malignant neoplasms and premalignant diseases which show classical mendelian inheritance patterns.

tion and adequate controls. However, since the 1930's and 40's these problems have been rectified to a large extent, and as a result much useful knowledge in the field of human cancer genetics has been obtained. Many syndromes in which cancer is integral have been described. In addition, a number of diseases have been shown to have an increased statistical association with malignant neoplasms.

During the past decades, increasing numbers of studies confirming and reconfirming patterns of mendelian inheritance for several premalignant disorders and for certain site specific cancers have appeared in the literature. Table 1 is a current listing of these conditions and their particular modes of inheritance. This list undoubtedly will increase as research in cancer genetics continues.

In addition to the conditions showing classical patterns of mendelian inheritance, a large number of malignant neoplasms exists in which a genetic etiology is probably manifested to a greater or lesser degree but its true significance remains unclear; similarly, a number of hereditary diseases are suspected of being precancerous but the significance of their cancer association is unclear. These conditions are listed in table 2.

In addition to the conditions mentioned in tables 1 and 2, several of the more common malignant neoplasms in man, specifically adenocarcinoma of the colon, stomach, breast and endometrium, show a definite hereditary predisposition with at least a threefold increased risk to relatives of the cancer proband. However, patterns of mendelian inheritance have not yet been identified for these lesions.

Finally, still another category of problems in cancer genetics, namely that of "cancer families" with a specific histologic variety of cancer, is of interest to the clinician. The study of cancer of multiple anatomic sites, with careful pathologic documentation of tumors, was first instituted by Warthin[3] in 1913 in his investigation of Family G. This pedigree was updated in 1925[4] and in 1936.[5] The pattern of inheritance as well as the variety and distribution of tumors in this kindred has continued to be perpetuated.[6] Studies of other cancer families have shown striking similarities to Warthin's original observations.[7-9] Recently, it has been suggested that the phenomenon of cancer families constitutes a hereditary syndrome with the following characteristics: (1) a high frequency of adenocarcinoma of all anatomic sites but with a particular predilection for adenocarcinoma of the colon and the endometrium; (2) a greater frequency of multiple primary malignant neoplasms than that found in the general population; (3) an early age at onset of carcinoma; and (4) apparent autosomal dominant inheritance.[10]

This report focuses attention upon the important application of clinical genetics to the cancer problem in man. Emphasis is placed upon the role of one phase of clinical genetics, namely genetic counseling, and its significance in early cancer diagnosis with specific reference to "cancer families."

Genetic Counseling

Figure 1 is the pedigree of a cancer family. Note the significant increase in cancer including a high incidence of multiple primary malignant neoplasms and a relatively early age at the onset of cancer. Obvious questions are: (1) What are the implications for early cancer detection? (2) How can genetic counseling be of help?

The answer to the first question is primarily the physician's awareness that he is dealing with a cancer family. He must appreciate the fact that cancer in such families will not appear in the characteristic manner which he customarily has observed in his medical training or practice. For example, cancer statistics based on the general population show that adenocarcinoma of the colon has its onset in the mid-fifties and endometrial carcinoma in

TABLE 2

Hodgkin's disease	Wilms' tumor
Waldenstrom's macroglobulinemia	Werner's syndrome
Multiple myeloma	Paget's disease (osteitus deformans) and osteogenic sarcoma
Leukemia	Dermatomyositis
Kaposi's sarcoma	Sjogren's syndrome
Carcinoma of the nasopharynx	Scleroderma (progressive systemic sclerosis)
Generalized keratoacanthoma (rare examples of malignant neoplasia)	Systemic lupus erythematosis
Hepatocellular carcinoma	Albinism
Pheochromocytoma	Dysgenetic gonads and disorders of somatosexual disturbance
Carcinoid tumor	
Carcinoma of the duodenum	Porphyria cutanea tarda
Testicular tumors	Intraocular melanoma
Neuroblastoma	Cutaneous melanoma

A listing of malignant neoplasms and premalignant diseases wherein either a hereditary etiology or predisposition to cancer is being investigated.

the late fifties and early sixties. However, both of these lesions occur 10 to 15 years earlier in cancer families. Similarly, multiple primary malignant neoplasms occur in about 2 to 5% of cancer patients in the general population. However, multiple primary malignant neoplasms occurred in over 19% of the members of cancer families.[11]

Finally, the physician must be cognizant of the significantly increased risk of cancer to relatives of his cancer family patients. This point is illustrated by the pedigree in figure

FIG. 1

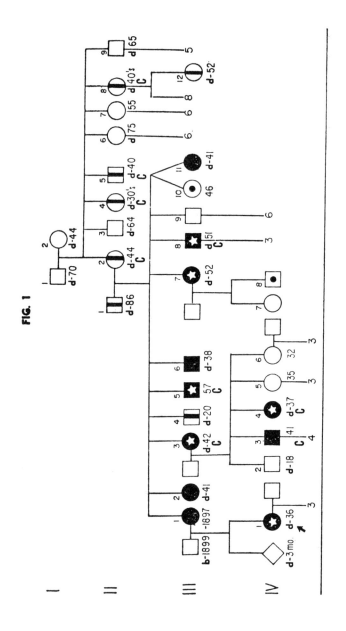

🖌 - PROBAND

d - DECEASED

PROGENY
6 NOT EXAMINED

6
☐ OR ◯ MALE OR FEMALE UNAFFECTED
REFERENCE NUMBER
32 AGE

■ OR ● " WITH HISTOLOGIC PROOF OF CANCER

▤ ⊖ " WITH CANCER BY HISTORY (NO HISTOLOGICAL PROOF)

★ ✪ " WITH TWO OR MORE PRIMARY MALIGNANT NEOPLASMS

⊙ ⊡ " WITH BENIGN TUMOR
C " WITH ADENOCARCINOMA OF COLON

Pedigree of a "cancer family" showing an increased occurrence of cancer, including **multiple primary malignant neoplasms** and an early age at onset of cancer. (Previously published in Arch Intern Med 117:209, 1966. **Permission granted for republication by editor.)**

59

1. When advising relatives from these families of their cancer risk, great care must be used not to alarm them, since this will only increase their apprehension, anxiety and fear, and perhaps will cause them to delay in seeking medical attention for early signs and symptoms of cancer.

The implications for genetic counseling are profound. Fear of a cancer diagnosis appears to be particularly prevalent and intensified in members of cancer families[12] as well as in relatives from families with other varieties of hereditary malignant diseases.[13] Emphasizing the positive aspects of early cancer diagnosis appears to be a good way of handling this problem. This involves early education of patients about cancer. This point is emphasized since we have often observed considerable apathy and fatalism in patients of cancer families, particularly in those who have observed the untoward effects of cancer among their relatives. Thus, it would seem that the earlier education in cancer is begun and a philosophy of cancer prevention is instilled in patients, the more likely will be the success in counteracting a complacent or fatalistic attitude about cancer.

A major objective in counseling patients with hereditary cancer is the alleviation of the patient's fears and anxieties. Since the anxiety which is provoked by the fear of cancer may cause the patient to be imprudent in his judgments and actions about cancer, the physician must be willing to take the time to listen to the patient and to encourage him to discuss openly his feelings, attitudes and fears about cancer. In our experience, such a catharsis may prove to be therapeutic to the patient by permitting him to achieve a more accurate understanding of the nature of the disease and its individual relationship to him.

Genetic facts about inheritance of cancer in the patient's family are discussed only when the physician believes that his patient is psychologically capable of coping with this material and effectively acting upon it. As a simple tool in genetic counseling, we teach the patient the fundamentals of pedigree construction, taking care to explain that the symbols used are merely a convenient way of talking about families. The basic rudiments of the biology of inheritance are discussed, with attention given to the patient's sophistication and educational background. It is interesting that patients with only meager formal education can readily comprehend this material. The patient then is encouraged to participate actively in the construction of his own family pedigree. We have found that this approach enables him to appraise the cancer problem in his family more objectively and promotes more acceptance of genetic risk factors for cancer.

The patient in a "cancer family" is advised of the apparent dominant pattern of inheritance. He is shown that the risk of receiving the cancer gene is approximately 50%, depending upon the medical history of his relatives. Conversely, the 50% chance of his not receiving the cancer gene is given equal emphasis. Since the cancer risk increases with age regardless of the patient's genetic background, he is encouraged to continue with a program of cancer detection throughout his life. The patient may accept this fact when he is shown the relatively high incidence of cancer in the general population and that, although he harbors an increased genetic risk for cancer, he is really no different from the average individual. Finally, genetic counseling can be used effectively by the physician for cancer education of relatives of his patient. The patient who can accept objectively an increased risk of cancer, and who recognizes the importance of early cancer detection, may become the physician's single best ally for promoting a more positive, constructive approach to the cancer problem in his family. Thus, case finding and cancer control in relatives at risk for the early development of cancer could be the reward.

These principles are equally applicable to patients with malignant neoplasms and premalignant disorders outlined in tables 1 and

2. The physician must use every means available to him in his medical armamentarium to diagnose cancer at significantly earlier stages. We believe that knowledge of hereditary factors in cancer coupled with the patience and faith required in genetic counseling can help immeasurably in attaining these goals.

Two additional clinical examples clearly illustrate this thesis.

Case Reports

(1) A study was made of a family which manifested familial polyposis coli, a disease which is inherited as an autosomal dominant. The proband was a 20 year old white woman who had a history of weight loss, intermittent diarrhea, and melena noted over a 3 month period. Her father died from carcinoma of the colon at age 30. Her 27 year old brother, following a diagnosis of multiple polyposis coli, had had a colectomy for adenocarcinoma in a polyp at the rectosigmoid junction when he was 23 years old.

On the basis of the clinical findings and her family history, the obvious diagnostic impression entertained for our patient was familial polyposis coli. In fact, this diagnosis became apparent within moments upon proctosigmoidoscopy examination. Unfortunately, she had an advanced adenocarcinoma of the colon. Had she been evaluated for this disease 4 years previously, at the time that this diagnosis was established in her brother, she undoubtedly could have been afforded a much more favorable prognosis through appropriate surgical treatment.

Her father probably also had polyposis coli although we were able to establish only the fact that he had adenocarcinoma of the colon. The father's early age at the manifestation of this disease and the fact that 2 of his children had polyposis coli are highly significant. The physician managing this family could have practiced effective preventive medicine and cancer control through calling the attention of responsible members of the family to the hereditary characteristics of this disease. In such an autosomal dominant disease, one could have predicted that approximately one-half of the father's children and one-half of his siblings would have inherited this disease (barring the possibility that this disease resulted from a mutation in one of his parents). Since virtually all patients with this condition develop cancer by age 50, the treatment is preventive in the form of a prophylactic colectomy once the diagnosis has been established unequivocally. The earlier this is performed, the less the risk for cancer transformation in one of the myriad polyps which carpet the colon of these patients. Genetic counseling, therefore, is directed toward all phases of the disease, i.e., case finding in relatives, diagnosis and therapy. Careful handling of emotional factors is also an essential part of cancer genetic counseling.

(2) In another example involving xeroderma pigmentosum (x.d.p.), a surgeon who was aware of the hereditary aspect of this disease was able to establish the diagnosis in 4 of the proband's 7 siblings. Implication for cancer control in the form of restriction of solar radiation for the affected youngsters was assiduously followed by the family. This has resulted in an unusually benign clinical course of the disease in this family. Through genetic counseling, we were able to correct many misconceptions about the inheritance of x.d.p. and to provide considerable reassurance to the family.[14] For example, 2 of the older sisters were fearful of marriage because they thought they might transmit the disease to their children. We were able to show them that the chance for this was negligible if they did not marry a close relative. Since the gene for x.p.d. is rare, it would be unlikely that they would marry someone homozygous (affected) or heterozygous (a carrier) for this gene. Considerable resolution of anxiety resulted and they have made excellent heterosexual adjustments.

Summary

Genetic counseling should be considered an integral part of the medical management of the patient with hereditary disease. This is even more important when dealing with life threatening diseases such as cancer. Physicians certainly are aware of the importance of genetic counseling but all too often have referred these problems to nonmedically trained geneticists. McKusick[1] has taken issue with this attitude; he believes that genetic counseling should be done more frequently by the physician who is closest to the patient's problem. He observed:

"Too long genetic counseling has, by default, fallen to the province of the college professor of genetics, who is informed that the diagnosis is Humpty Dumpty's disease, who looks up the usual mode of inheritance of H-D disease in a book and on the basis of this and the specific pedigree gives advice. Genetic counseling, like other medical prognoses, should be an integral part of the practice of clinical medicine. The physician is in the best position to meet (the patients needs for genetic counseling) . . . (and) with improved education in medical genetics sound genetic counseling should become the rule in medical practice."[1]

We subscribe wholeheartedly to this philosophy and think that the entire management of the complex cancer problem, including genetic counseling, should be under the physician's direction.

References

1. McKusick, V. A.: Genetics in Medicine and Medicine in Genetics, Amer J Med 4:594, 1963.
2. Lynch, H. T.: Hereditary Factors in Carcinoma, *Recent Results in Cancer Research*. Vol. 12. Berlin, Springer-Verlag, 1967, p. 186.
3. Warthin, A. S.: Heredity with Reference to Carcinoma as Shown by the Study of the Cases Examined in the Pathological Laboratory of the University of Michigan, 1895-1913, Arch Intern Med 12:546, 1913.
4. Warthin, A. S.: The Further Study of a Cancer Family, J Cancer Res 9:279, 1925.
5. Hauser, I. J., and Weller, C. W.: A Further Report on the Cancer Family of Warthin, Amer J Cancer 27:434, 1936.
6. Lynch, H. T.: Unpublished data, 1967.
7. Bieler, V., and Heim, U.: Doppelkarzinom Bei Geschwistern Familiäre Häufung Von Genital-und Intestinalkarzinomen, Schweiz Med Wschr 95:496, 1965.

8. Savage, D.: A Family History of Uterine and Gastrointestinal Cancer, Brit Med J 2:341, 1956.

9. Heinzelmann, N. F.: A Cancer Prone Family. Discussion of the Question of Inheritability of Colonic Carcinoma, Helv Chir Acta 31:316, 1964.

10. Lynch, H. T., Anderson, D. E., Krush, A. J., and Larsen, A. L.: Heredity and Carcinoma, Ann NY Acad Sci, in press.

11. Lynch, H. T., Krush, A. J., and Larsen, A. L.: Heredity and Multiple Primary Malignant Neoplasms: Six Cancer Families, Amer J Med Sci, 254:322, 1967.

12. Krush, A. J., Lynch, H. T., and Magnuson, C. W.: Attitudes Toward Cancer in a "Cancer Family": Implications for Cancer Detection, Amer J Med Sci 249:432, 1965.

13. Dukes, C. E.: Cancer Control in Familial Polyposis of the Colon, Dis Colon Rectum 1:413, 1928.

14. Lynch, H. T., Anderson, D. E., Smith, J. L., Howell, J. B., and Krush, A. J.: Xeroderma Pigmentosum, Malignant Melanoma, and Congenital Ichthyosis: A Family Study, Arch Derm (Chicago) 96:625, 1967.

Practical Aspects of the Family History, Genetics, and Genetics Counseling: Cancer

HENRY T. LYNCH, M.D.

KNOWLEDGE of the role of hereditary factors in malignant neoplasms could aid the physician in making an *early* diagnosis of cancer in patients and their relatives who might be genetically at risk. Figures released by the American Cancer Society indicate that approximately 300,000 Americans expired from cancer in 1966. Of these, approximately 95,000 could have been saved through *earlier* cancer diagnosis.[1] We believe that knowledge of the family history and the inheritance patterns of cancer, could lead to an early diagnosis in patients with an increased hereditary predisposition toward cancer.

In our experience, the family history is often severely neglected in patient evaluation, particularly in patients with cancer. Recently, this problem was discussed with hundreds of physicians, while displaying an exhibit on heredity a n d carcinoma at meetings of the American Medical Association,[2] many of whom expressed amazement that certain cancers could be considered hereditary.

In part, the lack of attention to the "family history" can be accounted for by the absence of formal courses in human genetics in many medical schools. Genetics is rarely a requirement for medical school; when formally offered in medical school, it frequently represents a very small proportion of the total curriculum. In short, the genetic aspects of disease receive insufficient attention in the training of physicians.

The purpose of this report is to provide a listing of malignant neoplasms and precancerous disorders which either show classical mendelian inheritance patterns or have an increased empiric risk of developing in close relatives of a proband.[3] In addition, comments will be made on genetic counseling, based on experience with a variety of diseases in over 700 families.[4-12]

Classical Examples of Hereditary Cancers (Table 1)

The role of hereditary factors in most malignant neoplasms of man is not clear. Nonhereditary factors undoubtedly have a part in many of these diseases. Several types of cancer and disorders predisposing to cancer have been identified as having classic mendelian inheritance patterns, and the number is increasing. It is essential to realize that classic mendelian inheritance does *not* exclude the possible contribution of extragenetic factors, *i.e.* possible carcinogens in man's environment such as oncogenic viruses, tobacco, ultraviolet radiation, smog, and hydrocarbons, which might be interacting with the genome in the production of cancer.[13] In addition, s o m e conditions (Table 1) may represent phenocopies, *i.e.* the disease may mimic the genetic variety, or a particular disorder may be manifested in certain families through mendelian inheritance and occur sporadically in the gen-. eral population. Some of these disorders could be caused by mutations; others may result from the influence of environmental carcinogens. Even in the latter situation, host factors may be of importance, although they are less critical than are environmental factors. A classical example is cancer of the urinary bladder, an occupational disease in workers in the dye industry resulting from chronic exposure to aniline dyes.

At present, there is no way of distinguishing either histologically or biochemically between malignant neoplasms which might be the result of strong hereditary influence and those which result primarily from environmental factors. A particular neoplasm may occur more frequently on a sporadic or so-called nongenetic basis; however, it may also be present with extremely high frequency in certain families. An example of this is *carotid body tumors.* These lesions are rare in the general population and occur most frequently on a sporadic basis. However, when occurring on a familial basis, they behave as classic autosomal dominants, affecting approximately 50 percent of the relatives and appearing often in multiple generations.[14]

When the diagnosis is established for any of the disorders listed in Table 1, the physician often can predict with mathematical probability the risk of development of malignant neoplasms in his patient's relatives. Further knowledge of the family history of a patient may greatly aid the physician in arriving at a diagnosis. An often cited and excellent example of this axiom is familial polyposis coli. The diagnosis of this disease, which often is caused by hereditary factors, will immediately indicate that either the patient's mother or his father was or is affected (assuming a mutation has not oc-

Table 1

Disorder	Inheritance
Familial polyposis coli	Autosomal dominant
Gardner's syndrome	" "
Hereditary exostosis	" "
Nevoid basal cell carcinoma syndrome	" "
Hereditary polyendocrine adenomatosis	" "
Medullary thyroid carcinoma with amyloid production and pheochromocytoma	" "
Peutz-Jeghers syndrome	" "
Tylosis (keratosis et palmaris plantaris) and esophageal cancer	" "
Von-Recklinghausen's neurofibromatosis	" "
Retinoblastoma	" "
Carotid body tumors	" "
Von-Hippel Lindau disease	" "
Tuberous sclerosis	" "
Xeroderma pigmentosum	Autosomal recessive
Bloom's syndrome	" "
Fanconi's aplastic anemia	" "
Ataxia telangiectasia (Louis-Bar syndrome)	" "
Chediak-Higashi syndrome	" "
Wiskott-Aldrich syndrome	" "
Sex-linked agammaglobulinemia (Bruton's type)	Sex-linked

This table lists malignant neoplasms and precancerous disorders in man showing classical mendelian inheritance patterns.

curred), and that approximately 50 percent of the patient's siblings and 50 percent of his progeny will also be be affected. Any patient w h o gives a family history of this disease should be carefully evaluated and all available tests, *i.e.* (proctosigmoidoscopy and barium enema) should be used to exclude the presence of polyposis of the colon. If the diagnosis is colonic polyposis, a colectomy must be performed as the risk of developing adenocarcinoma of the colon is extremely high. Without colectomy approximately 50 per cent of these patients will develop cancer by age 30 and virtually 100 per cent will do so by age 50.[15]

Common Malignant Neoplasms of Man and Heredity (Table 2)

Hereditary factors appear to be important in the etiology of several of the more frequently occurring malignant neoplasms in man. However, the specific mode of inheritance has not yet been delineated for any of the conditions cited in Table 2. The conditions may be the result of the interaction of genetic and environmental factors, *i.e.* genotypically susceptible individuals may have had insufficient exposure to carcinogens or other environmental factors (early death from other causes, etc.), or the magnitude of the environmental factors may obfuscate any genetic differences. Certainly, pertinent data substantiates this reasoning in cancer of the lung and breast. Tokuhata[16] found that patients who have a positive family history for cancer of the lung and who are heavy smokers have a risk 14 times greater than do patients with neither of these characteristics. Those who have the familial factor but who do *not* smoke, have a fourfold risk over those without the familial factor who do not smoke.

Macklin[17] has shown the importance of parity in addition to family background in patients with adenocarcinoma of the breast.

Table 2

Breast carcinoma	Endometrial carcinoma
Colon carcinoma	Prostate carcinoma
Stomach carcinoma	Lung carcinoma

This table lists the more common malignant neoplasms in man for which hereditary factors appear to be important but for which the mode of inheritance has not as yet been identified.

Nulliparous individuals showed a higher frequency of breast cancer than do their multiparous relatives. In general, first degree female relatives of breast cancer probands[4] have a threefold risk for development of carcinoma of the breast.

Miscellaneous Cancer and Cancer Predisposing Disorders (Table 3)

Geneticists and epidemiologists have given considerable attention to the conditions listed in Table 3 from the standpoint of inheritance and/or relationship to the development of malignant neoplasms. For example, albinism is usually inherited as an autosomal recessive trait and an increased frequency of malignant neoplasms, particularly squamous and basal cell carcinomas of the skin, appears to occur in this disorder. However, the significance of this relationship to development of cancer remains unclear. On the contrary, Kaposi's sarcoma and nasopharyngeal carcinoma show definite racial and possible geographic predilections, but the significance of hereditary and environmental factors in the disorders remains an enigma. These disorders pose a challenge which can be approached best through the

Table 3

Hodgkin's disease	Wilms' tumor
Waldenstrom's macroglobulinemia	Werner's syndrome
Multiple myeloma	Paget's disease (osteitis deformans) and osteogenic sarcoma
Leukemia	
Kaposi's sarcoma	Dermatomyositis
Carcinoma of the nasopharynx	Sjogren's syndrome
Generalized keratoacanthoma (rare examples of malignant neoplasia)	Scleroderma (progressive systemic sclerosis)
Hepatocellular carcinoma	Systemic lupus erythematosis

Pheochromocytoma_____Albinism	
Carcinoid tumor_____Dysgenetic gonads and disorders of somato-sexual disturbance	
Carcinoma of the duodenum_____Porphyria cutanea tarda	
Testicular tumors_____Intraocular melanoma	
Neuroblastoma_____Cutaneous melanoma	

This table lists malignant neoplasms and precancerous disorders of man wherein hereditary factors appear to be important. However, numerous epidemiologic factors appear to be interacting with the genome in these conditions posing a complex problem for genetic analysis.

combined efforts of geneticists and epidemiologists.

Meanwhile, some practical generalizations about these diseases can be considered. For example, a physician treating the Bantu of southwest Africa must be cognizant of the clinical presentation and pathology of Kaposi's sarcoma; in southwest Africa, this lesion is the most common malignant tumor of the upper and lower limbs.[18] Similarly, physicians who h a v e m a n y patients of Chinese and Malaysian extraction must be unusually alert to the occurrence of nasopharyngeal carcinoma. The mortality rate of immigrants from China from nasopharyngeal carcinoma is 30 to 40 times greater than is that for Caucasians.[19] The mortality rate from nasopharyngeal cancer in Chinese born in the United States is 20 times that for Caucasians.[19]

"Cancer Families"

"Cancer families," as we have defined them, have the following characteristics: (1) an increased frequency of adenocarcinomas (the most common are those of the colon and endometrium); (2) an increased frequency of multiple primary malignant neoplasms; and (3) an earlier age at onset for these malignant neoplasms as opposed to the occurrence of the same histologic variety in the general population. Autosomal dominant inheritance appears to be the most likely explanation, though further study will be necessary to confirm this.[20] The frequency of occurrence of this phenomenon in the population is not known.

The physician must be prepared to find a variety of malignant neoplasms in "cancer families." Should he make a diagnosis of cancer, the physician should continue to search for additional malignant neoplasms. In short, cancer-prone individuals from these families should be followed closely and given frequent cancer detection tests. Evaluations should be started at earlier ages than usual, and patients should be considered cancer-susceptible throughout their lives. Psychological management must be a major part of the plan as it is in all cancer problems.

General Considerations

The application of genetic knowledge to the early diagnosis of human diseases has assumed considerable importance in several of the autosomal recessive enzymatic deficiency disorders, including phenylketonuria, maple syrup urine disease, and galactosemia. In this group of diseases, an early diagnosis followed promptly by dietary management can significantly alter the prognosis. A similar situation applies for certain human cancers. Genetic knowledge in these instances can bring early diagnosis with significant improvement in prognosis through prompt management of the precancerous or cancer problem. Knowledge of the role of heredity in carcinoma, securing a thorough family history, and genetic counseling, can help improve the prognosis of patients with hereditary cancer.

Recent origin and limited use preclude the full development of a philosophy of genetic counseling. In our philosophy, genetic counseling becomes as much a part of total patient management as the medical history, physical examination, laboratory studies, and therapeutic plan. This is particularly true in patients with certain types of cancer and other hereditary life threatening diseases, since the goal of genetic counseling is not only to provide the patient with accurate genetic risk information at a time when he is psychologically able to handle this material, but also to encourage continuous communication between the physician and the family for more expedient management of the "family disease." When the physician lacks knowledge of the hereditary factors involved in a particular disorder, he can refer the family to a medical genetics clinic. Most such clinics serve primarily in a consultant capacity, with research and service to the family as the primary objectives. A constant feedback to the family physician is thus established, with the family unit receiving the maximum benefit.

We have been impressed with the profound emotional overtones present in many patients with "family diseases," particularly those with disorders which are disfiguring to the body[21] or result in early death.[5] In counseling such patients, the physician must be cognizant of occasionally intense emotional responses of these individuals to the "family disease," which may cause them to repress or deny it in themselves or their relatives; some patients may be apathetic and others may be frankly hostile. Communication may be difficult and remarks made by the physician often may be grossly distorted.

Accurate diagnosis is essential and is often easier when the physician fully appreciates the range of expression which hereditary disease may show. For example, a patient with blue sclerae but no history of bone fractures or with a hearing deficiency and a family history of osteogenesis imperfecta should be considered affected. Fifty percent of his children will have a risk of developing either mild or severe osteogenesis imperfecta. Similarly, the presence of *cafe au lait* spots (particularly when these are in the axillae) with otherwise normal findings in a patient with a family history of neurofibromatosis indicates the *forme fruste* of the disease. In other words, the patient harbors the gene for this disorder, in which the genetic risks are similar to those for osteogenesis imperfecta. Moreover, this individual harbors an increased risk for the development of malignant neoplasms, particularly acoustic neuromas (most often bilateral), meningiomas, and gliomas. Genetic counseling should, therefore, embrace the total clinical picture, which includes diagnosis and dissemination of accurate genetic risk information, but only when the patient is psychologically *ready* to accept and understand. In our experience with cancer patients, the problem may be compounded further by either profound *fear* or *apathy* and *fatalism* toward a diagnosis of cancer. In any event, a *delay* in cancer diagnosis may be an unfortunate consequence. Much of the emotional reaction to carcinoma has been fostered by misconceptions which often cause patients to exaggerate the disease's seriousness; many view cancer as incurable, with a uniformly hopeless prognosis. This impression may be further tempered by the attitudes and feelings of the physician who may also reflect a negative attitude toward cancer.[22] The physician may be completely unaware of his "hopeless" approach to his cancer patients and their families; however, this feeling is often fully transmitted to these individuals. More can be gained from the standpoint of *earlier* c a n c e r diagnosis through offering as bright and *positive* picture as is honestly possible. The *cure* potential that can be offered the patient through early diagnosis should be emphasized. Again, familial polyposis coli, can be used as an example. This condition should not be dreaded and considered "hopeless;" if diagnosed sufficiently early, it can be cured in virtually 100 percent of the patients through removal of the diseased colon. On the basis of his long experience with familial polyposis coli, Dukes[22] has emphasized the value of a matter-of-fact approach to his patients, beginning in the *early teens* and using routine follow-up studies. The positive aspect of *cure* through early diagnosis should be constantly emphasized. In our studies of cancer genetic problems, we have found this philosophy successful.

Summary

Malignant neoplasms a n d premalignant disorders of man which are known or suspected to have a genetic etiology have been cited. Practical application of this knowledge in *earlier* cancer diagnosis in the *patient* and his *relatives* has been stressed. Guidelines toward genetic counseling in hereditary cancer problems have been discussed.

Physicians certainly are aware of the importance of genetic counseling but all too often have referred these problems to nonmedically trained geneticists. McKusick[23] has taken issue with this attitude; he feels that genetic counseling should be performed more frequently by the physician who is closest to the patient's problem. He observed:

"Too long genetic counseling has, by default, fallen to the province of the college professor of genetics, who is informed that the diagnosis is Humpty Dumpty's disease, who looks up the usual mode of inheritance of H-D disease in a book and on the basis of this and the specific pedigree gives advice. Genetic counseling, like other medical prognosis, should be an integral part of the practice of clinical medicine. The physician is in the best position to meet (the patient's needs for genetic counseling) . . . (and) with improved education in medical genetics sound genetic counseling should become the rule in medical practice."

We have formulated ten so called "commandments" for effective genetic counseling as follows:

1. Genetic counseling is an integral part of the management of the patient with genetic disease, the responsibility for which ideally should be assumed by the family physician.

2. The counselor must never make decisions for the patient regarding marriage, children, and other important personal issues. These decisions are the patient's responsibility and only he should exercise this right.

3. The genetic counselor must take meticulous care to insure the accuracy of diagnosis in hereditary disease in that ramifications of such a diagnosis may profoundly affect the entire family unit.

4. The counselor must look beyond his individual patient and be concerned with eliciting support for the medical welfare of other affected members of the kindred.

5. The genetic counselor must constantly remember that the presence of hereditary diseases in the family may promote strong emotional reaction among affected as well as unaffected members of the kindred; the

counselor, must do everything possible to alleviate this emotional stress.

6. The genetic counselor must strive effectively to dispel unfavorable impressions and irrational responses by members of the community against individuals with certain grotesque mental and physical hereditary disorders. The physician will usually be in a favorable position in the community to institute a positive educational program toward this goal.

7. The genetic counselor must study all aspects of the natural history of hereditary diseases, so that when needed he may effectively mobilize paramedical personnel and community resources to help the patient and his family.

8. Care must be taken to exclude extra genetic factors as being of etiologic importance. Should a nongenetic factor be the major cause of disease, i.e., rubella syndrome, parents must be reassured and thoroughly informed that the disorder in their midst is not genetic, should this be the case.

9. Hearsay evidence of disease in relatives of the affected proband should be verified whenever possible; effort extended in this direction will in the long run be highly rewarding.

10. The genetic counselor will be in a favorable position to study variations in known hereditary disorders as well as to uncover "new" hereditary diseases. He should make every effort to report his scientific observations to his colleagues.

References
1. American Cancer Society: Cancer Facts and Figures, American Cancer Society, New York, 1966.
2. Lynch, T. T.; Anderson, D. E., and Krush, A. J.: Heredity and carcinoma: A study of cancer families. Exhibit presented to the Annual Meeting of the American Medical Association, June 26-30,

1966, Chicago, Illinois, and to the Clinical Sessions of the American Medical Association, Las Vegas, Nevada, November 27 - December 1, 1966.

3. Lynch, H. T.: Hereditary Factors in Carcinoma. Springer - Verlag, Berlin, Germany, 1967, pp. 186.

4. Lynch, H. T., and Krush, A. J.: Heredity and breast cancer: Implications for cancer control. Med Times 94:599, 1966.

5. Lynch, H. T.; Krush, T. P., and Krush, A. J.: Psychodynamics in cancer detection: A patient with advanced cancer of the lip. Psychosomatics 7:152, 1966.

6. Lynch, H. T.; Krush, T. P.; Krush, A. J., and Tips, R. L.: Psychodynamics of early hereditary deaths. Amer J Dis Child 108:605, 1964.

7. Lynch, H. T.; Tips, R. L.: Krush, A. J., and Magnuson, C. W.: Family centered genetic counseling and the medical genetics clinic. Nebraska Med J 50:155, 1965.

8. Krush, A. J.; Lynch, H. T., and Magnuson, C. W.: Attitudes toward cancer in a "cancer family:" Implications for cancer detection. Amer J Med Sci 249:432, 1965.

9. Tips, R. L.; Smith, G. S.; Lynch, H. T., and McNutt, C. W.: The "whole family" concept in clinincal genetics. Amer J Dis Child 107:67, 1964.

10. Tips, R. L., and Lynch, H. T.: The impact of genetic counseling upon the family milieu. JAMA 184:183, 1963.

11. Lynch, H. T.; Anderson, D. E.; Krush, A. J., and Mukerjee, D.: Cancer, heredity, and genetic counseling: Xeroderma pigmentosum. Cancer, in press.

12. Lynch, H. T., and Krush, A. J.: Heredity, emotions, and cancer control. Postgrad Med, in press.

13. Lillienfeld, A. M.: Formal discussion of: Genetic factors in the etiology of cancer: An epidemiologic view. Cancer Res 24:1330, 1965.

14. Resler, D. R.; Snow, J. B., and Williams, G. R.: Multiplicity and familial incidence of carotid body and glomus jugulare tumors. Ann Otol 75:114, 1966.

15. Dockerty, M.D.: Pathologic aspects in the control of spread of colonic carcinoma. Mayo Clin Proc 33:157, 1958.

16. Tokuhata, G. K.: Familial factors in human lung cancer and smoking. Amer J Public Health 54:24, 1964.

17. Macklin, M.: Relative status of parity and genetic background in producing human breast cancer. J Nat Cancer Inst 23:1179, 1959.

18. Oettle, A.: Geographical and racial differences in the frequency of Kaposi's sarcoma as evidence of environmental or genetic cancer. Acta un int cancr 18:330, 1962.

19. Buell, P.: Nasopharynx cancer in Chinese in California. Brit J Surg 19:459, 1965.

20. Lynch, H. T.; Shaw, M. W.; Magnuson, C. W.; Larsen, A. L., and Krush, A. J.: Hereditary

factors in cancer: Study of two large midwestern kindreds.   Arch Intern Med 117:206, 1966.

21.   Krush, A. J.; Krush, T. P., and Lynch, H. T.:   Psycho-social factors in a family with a disfiguring genetic fault.   Psychosomatics 6:391, 1965.

22.   Dukes, C. E.:   Familial intestinal polyposis. Ann Roy Coll Surg Eng 10:293-304, 1952.

23.   McKusick, V. A.:   Genetics in medicine and medicine in genetics.   Amer J Med 4:594, 1963.

TUBEROUS SCLEROSIS:
A CLINICAL AND GENETICAL INVESTIGATION*

J. ZAREMBA

Tuberous sclerosis (T.S.) consists of congenital developmental malformations affecting all three embryonic layers with particular predisposition for the organs developing from the ectoderm. It is characterised by the presence of tuberous nodes of almost any organs, but occurring most frequently in the skin, brain, retina, heart and kidneys. The nodes form as a result of disturbances in maturation and migration of individual cells in early embryonic life and exhibit but slight tendency to malignant growth.

Mental deficiency, epilepsy and Pringle's tumours form the most characteristic symptom triad which may, however, be manifest in a wide variety of forms according to the intensity and localisation of the lesions.

Various terms have been applied to the disease, such as tuberous sclerosis (Bourneville, 1880), Bourneville's disease or syndrome, Bourneville's phakomatosis (van der Hoeve, 1923), Pringle's disease and several others. Epiloia (Sherlock, 1911) occurs almost exclusively in the English literature.

T.S. belongs to the group of conditions known as phakomatoses ("dysplasies neuro-éctodermiques" of Van Bogaert, 1935 and "congenital ectodermoses" or "neurocutaneous syndromes" of Yakovlev and Guthrie, 1931) which have in common developmental malformations, and usually, dominant inheritance. The possibility should not be overlooked, however, that similar conditions may occur in the embryopathies. Besides T.S., the group includes Von Recklinghausen's disease, Hippel-Lindau disease, Sturge-Weber disease and the related Klippel-Trénaunay-Weber disease. Possibly, also, the so-called "fifth phakomatosis" syndrome which includes cysts: of the jaw, multiple naevoid basal cell carcinomata, developmental anomalies of vertebrae and ribs and brain and eye changes, should be included (Hermans, *et al.*, 1965). It has also been suggested (Waardenburg, 1963; Loesch, *et al.*, 1966) that neurocutaneous melanoblastosis, a term due to Touraine (1955) belongs to this group.

Tuberous sclerosis probably occurs in all races (Cornée and Le Bras, 1964; Randazzo and Greppi, 1964; Shinfuku and Kadowski, 1962) and typical lesions have recently been described in the brain of the rhesus monkey (Von Unterharnscheidt, 1964). An extensive survey of the literature by Vaas (1940) indicates similar incidence in both sexes.

The present investigation of 40 cases is a clinico-genetical one. It has not been our intention to contribute to symptomatology in general, but to verify on a large sample the incidence of particular symptoms or lesions, especially to establish their

* This work constitutes part of a doctor's thesis, June 1966 (not published), supported by grant of Children's Bureau, Department of Health, Education and Welfare, U.S.A., POL WA-CB-6.

Table 1

Ascertainment of cases

Classification	Source	Number		Sporadic	Familial
Propositi	in 23 institutions	19	⎫	15	11
	in hospital, Pruszków	7	⎬ 26		
Relatives of propositi	in 23 institutions	1	⎫	0	14
	out patients	13	⎬ 14		
Total cases studied			40	15	25
Extra case used for estimations only	in 23 institutions		1	—	—

usefulness in the diagnosis of abortive cases, since the ascertainment of subjects in whom the disease is only slightly manifest is of crucial importance for the genetic study. In the genetical part of the study we tried :

1. To detect the transmission of the T.S. gene in the particular pedigrees, that is to say, to make an attempt to solve the still not very clear, problem of penetration in this disease.

2. To estimate its incidence in the general population of Poland.

3. On the basis of detailed clinical examination, to evaluate what part of the material was composed of familial cases and what of sporadic ones.

4. On the basis of our conclusion to estimate the mutation rate of tuberous sclerosis.

MATERIAL AND METHODS

Twenty-three Polish institutions for severely retarded children aged 3-18 years were surveyed, with a total population of 1,887 (1,080 girls and 807 boys). The examination of this material revealed 20 propositi with T.S. (one extra subject was only included in estimating incidence). Seven other propositi were ascertained in the Pruszkow State Hospital for Nervous and Mental Diseases and in the genetic department of the Psychoneurological Institute. The remaining 14 cases were relatives of the propositi.

Ascertainment of the cases is presented in table 1.

There was thus a total of 40 cases in 26 families, 29 female and 11 male. No conclusions about sex incidence were drawn because of bias in the institutional populations, possibly due to the higher incidence of epilepsy in the females increasing the risk of admission.

Table 2

Frequency of the particular skin changes in 40 cases of T.S.

Pringle's tumours	Shagreen skin	Koenen's tumours	Depigmented naevi	Sessile fibromas
36	19	22	31	28

Pedunculated fibromas	Café au lait spots	Pigmented naevi	Angiomas	Fibromas of gums
6	6	2	1	22

Subjects were divided into 25 severe (idiots and imbeciles) and 15 mild and abortive, the mental level being the principle of division.

Patients in hospital were subjected to the following investigations: X-rays of skull, hands, feet and chest and urography; E.E.G., E.C.G.; chromosome analysis and routine laboratory tests. Most of them, and the relatives, were given mental tests. Relatives, 116 of whom were examined, received neurological examinations and usually E.E.G. recordings and X-rays. All fundi were examined with dilated pupils.

For genetical purposes, among the total of 26 families (15 without and 11 with evidence of transmission) there were 26 propositi and 14 secondary cases. The clinical division was also of genetical significance in so far as the severe group was biologically unfit, having a fertility value of zero, the mild group being fairly fit in this respect.

An attempt was made to analyse the manifestation of various symptoms within pedigrees. The major genetical part of this investigation however, has been the estimation of the mutation rate.

The possibility of a parental age effect has also been examined.

RESULTS

Clinical Findings

Skin changes (Table 2). Pringle's tumours were the commonest skin lesion in our material (90 per cent). These tumours are often small and barely discernible and and consequently easily missed. In 16 instances the parents did not notice the presence of these lesions on themselves and/or on their children. The average age of 16 patients when skin changes were observed by members of the family was 4.3 years, with a range of 1 to 8 years.

Second in frequency of occurrence was the depigmented naevus, in 31 subjects (77.5 per cent). It is less pathognomonic that Pringle's naevus, Koenen's tumours or shagreen skin, but nevertheless was seldom noted in the total number of unaffected children examined. In a group of 1,013 children examined in institutions for the severely retarded we found 109 with café-au-lait spots (10.8 per cent) and 33 with depigmented naevi (3.3 per cent). They are, therefore, of considerable diagnostic value in T.S., especially in abortive cases and for

102288

the detection of disease in relatives of propositi. It is worthy of note that depigmented naevi are present from birth, whereas Pringle's tumours and other skin lesions often do not appear earlier than the fourth of fifth year or life. The appearance and location of depigmented naevi is characteristic. They are discrete, usually oval in shape and metameric in distribution. On the trunk, distribution is transverse, on the limbs it is longitudinal. If present on hairy skin, the hairs are devoid of pigment.

Eye changes. Phakomata of the fundi were found in 19 subjects (47.5 per cent), in 8 of 15 slight and 11 of 25 severe cases, often bilaterally. It is of diagnostic value, particularly in abortive cases, sometimes being present in the absence of Pringle's tumours (3 cases). They tend to enlarge in the course of time and therefore are more commonly observed in adults than children. The size varies from a millet seed to a tumour larger than the optic disc. One subject had optic atrophy.

Neurological symptoms. Minor neurological symptoms are commonly encountered, particularly central paresis of the facial nerve (23 cases, 57.5 per cent), nystagmus 8 cases (20 per cent), signs of pyramidal involvement without paresis (24 cases, 60 per cent). Only in two, the paralysis of the form of spastic diplegia was found.

Microcephaly was found five times, enlargement of the skull due to hydrocephalus in two subjects. In one, on the side of the hemisphere more affected (contralateral spastic signs), the skull bones were less developed resulting in a pronounced asymmetry of the skull. The examination of CSF was performed in 18 cases. Changes in the form of mild pleocytosis were found only once.

Mental development. The mental level is shown in Table 3. Twenty four (60 per cent) are severely affected. The proportion of idiots to imbeciles in institutional patients with T.S. is 9 : 2, whereas the proportion for the remainder of the studied

Table 3

Mental level of subjects

Mental level	normal	feeble minded	imbeciles	idiots	Total
No.	12	4	5	19	40
%	30	10	12.5	47.5	100

Table 4

Age at onset of epilepsy in years

Age	1 1-6 mths.	7-12 mths.	2	3	4	5	6	7	8	9	10	>20	Total
Number	14	6	4	2	2	0	0	1	0	0	1	3	33

institutional population of 1887 is approximately 1 : 1 respectively. There are, however, 16 out of 40 total affected subjects mentally normal and only mildly afflicted, indicating that the condition tends to be mild or severe, with few intermediate cases. This is confirmed by examining sibs of propositi, including assessments from the available history of subjects who had died. (Four idiots, four normal and one borderline).

Epilepsy. Epilepsy occurred in 33 of 40 subjects. All propositi had fits at some time, those free of fits being exclusively members of their families. The onset was usually early (Table 4). The commonest type of seizure is the grand-mal attack, 18 instances (54.5 per cent). Judging from a detailed history, there were at least 13 examples (39 per cent) of infantile spasms. Other kinds of seizure, such as petit-mal, focal seizures and psychomotor attacks were also observed.

In seven patients the spontaneous regression of epilepsy was noted. The average period free of seizures in these patients was 14.3 years with a range of 6–30 years. In two members of families of affected subjects, epileptic fits occurred. However, in the absence of other signs of the disease, they were not considered as diagnostic. There was a tendency for early onset and more frequent fits to be associated with severe mental retardation.

E.E.G. Electroencephalography was undertaken in 32 patients with tuberous sclerosis and in 46 apparently unaffected relatives. Twelve of 32 tuberous sclerotics had normal tracings. Of 20 patients with abnormal E.E.G. records 14 exhibited generalized paroxysmal changes. In the group of 18 severely affected patients (all with seizures) there were two without E.E.G. changes. Only 4 of 14 mildly affected patients exhibited changes in E.E.G. tracings. These observations indicate that, like epilepsy, electroencephalograms are of limited diagnostic value in T.S.

Radiography. Thirty-four patients and 36 members of their families were investigated. The most common X-ray changes are presented in Table 5. No significant difference was found in radiological appearances of severe compared with mild and abortive cases (A and B). However, mild and abortive subjects tended to be older and it is well known that radiological changes of this kind may increase with age. X-ray changes were frequent and varied, the most useful films being of the skull, including air encephalography, and of the hands and feet. Lung cysts, of honeycomb appearance, were certainly present in only one out of 29 chest films. In 14 successful urographic films one renal tumour, one instance of double ureters and renal pelvices, one of suspected hydronephrosis and one of torsion of the kidney (possibly associated with scoliosis and torsion of the thoraco-lumber portion of the vertebral column) were found. There was also one example of a diverticulum in the wall of the bladder.

In most instances, radiological examination confirmed a previously established diagnosis. Only once did it resolve a doubtful diagnosis.

Occasional Clinical Findings. Asymmetry was observed occasionally, for instance of the face, hypertrophy of one great toe, hypertrophy of the soft tissues of one thumb and asymmetry of the lower extremities. Lateral distortion of the vertebral column was encountered in 8 subjects.

Table 5

Radiography findings in patients with tuberous sclerosis

Degree of disease	X-Ray of Skull					Pneumoencephalography				
		Intracranial calcification		Changes in cranial bones			Ventricular wall tumours ("candle guttering")		Internal hydro- cephalus	
	No. Ex- amined	No.	%	No.	%	No. Ex- amined	No.	%	No.	%
Mild and abortive	14	10	71.4	10	71.4	1	1	100	—	—
Severe	20	14	70.0	16	80.0	16	15	93.7	8	50.0
Total	34	24	70.6	26	75.5	17	16	94.1	8	47.0

X-Ray of Hands and Feet

	No. Examined Hands Feet		Cortical thickening of phalanges				Pseudocysts			
			Hands No. %		Feet No. %		Hands No. %		Feet No. %	
Mild and abortive	14	13	10	71.4	6	46.1	11	78.6	5	38.5
Severe	19	19	17	89.5	5	26.3	16	84.2	7	36.8
Total	33	32	27	81.8	11	34.4	27	81.8	12	37.5

E.C.G. recordings in 14 subjects revealed minor changes in two and did not appear to be of diagnostic value.

The analysis of karyotypes carried out in 9 cases didn't show any abnormality.

Genetical Analysis

For this purpose, the material consists of 40 affected subjects in 26 families. We have employed Weinberg's proband and sibship methods for estimating genetic ratios (Weinberg, 1912). The former is based on the formula :

$$P = \frac{R-N}{T-N}$$

where P is the genetic ratio, R, the total number of affected subjects, N, the number of families and T, the total number of offspring. Applied to our material, this gives :

$$P = \frac{30-24}{93-24} = 1 : 11.5$$

The formula for the sib method is :

$$P = \frac{r/r-1/}{r/s-1/}$$

where r is the number of affected sibs and s, the total number of sibs.

Our data gives :

$$P = \frac{16}{82} = 1 : 5$$

The values obtained are not compatible with any known type of inheritance, suggesting that our material cannot be treated as homogeneous. For instance, fresh mutations might be important in the occurrence of sporadic disease. We have therefore divided our material into familial and isolated cases for further analysis.

Familial Cases (Table 6). These consist of 11 propositi and 14 affected relatives, who were examined.

Estimation of the genetic ratio (affected : total sibs) in this group by the proband method gives 1 : 3.2. Bearing in mind that the method gives the minimal estimate, the deviation from the expected ratio of dominant inheritance is not great. The ratio obtained by the sibship method, however, is 1 : 2.4, which agrees fairly well with expectation. (The proportion of affected to unaffected sibs, excluding two families with an only child, was 15 : 13). Furthermore, the following observations indicate dominant transmission :

1. In each case, one parent was diseased, diagnosis being made by clinical examination in all but one instance, in which it was suggested by the history.
2. In no instance were the parents related.

High penetrance is supported by the absence of skipping of generations which occurs with incomplete penetrance. In one family the disease was observed in three

Table 6
Data of Familial Cases

Propositus No.	Sex of propositus	Number of affected in sibship	Sibs unaffected*	Stillbirths and abortions	Sex of affected parent	Parental age at birth of propositus (bold type) and of affected sibs		No. of generations in which the disease was detected
						father	mother	
3/III	F	3	2	3	M	27, 35, **41**	17, 25, **31**	3
7/V	F	2	—	—	M	23, **24**	22, **23**	3
11/VII	M	1	1	2	F	**28**	**27**	3
15/IX	F	1	3 (1)	—	M	**28**	**25**	2
16/X	M	3	2 (2)	2	F	47, **50**, 54	31, **34**, 38	2
21/XII	F	1	—	—	M	**33**	**24**	2
24/XIV	F	1	1	—	F	**35**	**28**	2
27/XVII	F	1	1	—	F	**22**	**22**	2
31/XIX	F	2	1	—	M	**26**, 29	**24**, 27	2
34/XXI	F	1	—	—	F	**26**	**29**	2
39/XXVI	F	1	2	—	F	**38**	**36**	2
Total		17	13	7	Mean	33.3	27.2	

*The figures given in brackets in column IV pertain to the sibs without symptoms of T.S. which died under 2 years of age. These were not taken into account in estimating genetic ratios.

generations and in two others disease in three generations was suggested by the family history. In the others, on the basis of clinical examination and of history, it seemed justifiable to assume its occurrence in two generations only, indicating rapid elimination of disease as a result of reduced fitness a finding which apparently accords with the intensification of disease with transmission observed in this material. We found one example only of a patient with a higher I.Q. than that of her affected parent (mother).

Our material is not sufficient to cover all aspects of hereditary transmission. In regard to severity, there are four possibilities of transmission : mild to severe, severe to mild, mild to mild and severe to severe. The second and the fourth may be neglected since zero fertility precludes them and the third could not be examined since our method of ascertainment introduced bias in favour of severely affected propositi. It is probably uncommon, however, as otherwise the incidence of T.S., particularly the abortive form known as Pringle's disease, would be much higher than it is. The present material consists almost exclusively of the first type of transmission and therefore does not permit general conclusions about intensification of disease in successive generations.

Isolated Cases. Details of the 15 examples of sporadic disease in our data (Table 7) include 5 families in which cases other than the propositi were classified as suspected on clinical grounds or on the evidence of history. Of these, the most controversial is Family IV, in which it may be that the father may have the gene and manifestation is slight. The sensitivity of our criteria of classification, however, is supported by the fact that in all our familial cases in which disease has been established in more than one sib, it has also been observed in one parent.

Propositi with apparently sporadic disease in our data may be of three origins : 1. Of families in which there are undetected abortive cases in relatives (possibly those marked with a question mark in Table 7). 2. Although improbable, some sporadic cases could be phenocopies. The mother of Propositus No. 26/XVI for instance was X-rayed several times in early pregnancy and was intensively treated for pulmonary tuberculosis. 3. Most sporadic examples of disease are likely to be the consequence of fresh mutations.

Incidence of Tuberous Sclerosis. The institutional component of our sample consisted of 21 patients ascertained between 1963 and 1965, in institutions for severely retarded children in the age range of 3–18 years. The children of this population were all severely or moderately retarded (idiot and imbecile level) and numbered 1,887 persons. The incidence of tuberous sclerosis within this population was therefore 1.1 per cent. The incidence of severe mental subnormality in the relevant age groups in Poland is 0.4 per cent (Wald and Stomma, 1965) which gives an incidence of $11/1,000 \times 4/1,000 = 1/22,727$, or 44×10^{-6}. This value may be somewhat elevated by the rather high proportion of epileptics in this population (about 30 per cent), since patients with T.S. occur more frequently amongst severely subnormal epileptics.

89

Table 7

Isolated and suspected cases

Propositus No.	Sex of the propositus	No. of sibs unaffected*	Stillbirths and Abortions	Birth rank of the propositus	Parental age at birth of the propositus father	mother
1/I	F	4		3	25	28
2/II	F	3 (1)		4	37	31
5/IV(?)	F	6		6	49	41
10/VI	F	2		3	36	32
13/VIII(?)	M	4		2	30	22
20/XI(?)	F	1		2	25	18
22/XIII	F	5	1	3	35	34
25/XV	F	1		2	31	21
26/XVI	F	1	1	1	26	21
29/XVIII	F	2 (1)		2	30	23
32/XX	F	10 (1)	1	11	48	44
35/XXII(?)	M	2 (1)		1	31	24
36/XXIII(?)	M	3		4	34	27
37/XXIV	F	1 (2)		3	26	32
38/XXV	M	8 (1)		3	31	27
Total		53			Mean 32.9	28.3

*The figures given in brackets in column III pertain to the sibs without symptoms of T.S. which died under 2 years of age, not taken into account in estimating genetic ratios.

90

Mutation Rate. The material examined for this purpose consisted of 15 sporadic and 11 familial propositi, 26 families in all. If the five families in which there was doubtful evidence of a familial tendency are excluded, there remain almost equal numbers of familial and sporadic propositi. It may therefore be estimated that in approximately half the families T.S. was the consequence of a fresh mutation. The mutation rate per person would then be $44 \times 10^{-6} \times 1/2$. The mutation rate is generally expressed, however, not per person, but per gene locus, since there are two gene loci (one on each homologous chromosome) per person at either of which a mutation may occur, and therefore the above figure corresponds to the double risk of mutation occurring at one or other gene locus. The estimated mutation rate as rate per gene locus i.e. per chromosome for tuberous sclerosis in our data is therefore $44 \times 10^{-6} \times 1/2 \times 1/2 = 11 \times 10^{-6}$. This corresponds to 11 mutations per generation in a population of half a million.

This value may seem to be too high because, as mentioned above, it is based on the incidence found in a population with a rather high frequency of epileptic subjects. However, reports in the literature (Berg and Crome, 1963; Borberg, 1951; Gunther and Penrose, 1935) and the present material (particularly if one includes suspected cases in the isolated group) suggest that actually T.S. may occur as a fresh mutation in more than half the families in which it is detected, so the estimate may be correct. Moreover, as our estimate was derived from severe cases, the true value may well be higher. One must take into consideration that mutations leading to severe disease, owing to the very low values of fitness, are elimated practically within one generation whereas those with mild manifestation give rise to familial cases, but even then, as our data show, they are not likely to survive for more than three generations. Therefore, assuming genetical equilibrium, in every generation the mutations of mild manifestation would have to arise to fill the deficit of one third of the families from which the gene of T.S. has been eliminated.

Familial occurrence of T.S. was observed in half of the families. Thus based upon the assumption of elimination of the T.S. gene in three generations, one can expect that in every generation from $1/3$ of this half, i.e. from $1/6$ of the total the gene of T.S. is eliminated and replaced by the corresponding number of the mild mutations which form a potential source of the new familial cases.

Therefore in every generation the proportion of cases due to fresh mutation would be by $1/6$ higher than originally found i.e. $1/2 + 1/6 = 2/3$. This would justify a correction to the previous estimate* : $44 \cdot 10^{-6} \cdot 2/3 \cdot 1/2 = 14.6 \cdot 10^{-6}$.

Against this one would claim that T.S. may be inherited in some families in mild form through many generations. We have, however, come to the conclusion (see "Familial cases") that such instances are rare, and the number of mutations required for their persistance would be negligible.

---

* Different estimates vary, being based on different assumptions. Penrose, for instance, originally estimated the mutation rate in T.S. as 8×10^{-6} per generation per locus. Further, he introduced a correction based on a different assumption from ours (above), but obtained a similar result : 12.5×10^{-6} (Penrose, 1936).

It is relevant to mention the frequent appearance in patients and their families of various developmental anomalies. No conclusion however can be drawn here without statistical analysis of larger material and without comparison with a proper control group.

Parental Age at Birth of Sporadic Cases. On the hypothesis that the older the parent the longer the risk period for the action of mutagenic agents, some late parental age effect might be expected. Raised mean paternal age at birth has been observed in chondrodystrophy (Grebe, 1955) and acrocephalosyndactyly (Grebe cit. according to Penrose, 1956) and raised maternal age is well-established in Down's syndrome.

No such effect is demonstrable in our material. Mean parental ages were calculated separately for sporadic (Table 7 and 8B) and familial subjects (Table 6 and 8A) and have been compared (Table 8) with the corresponding values for Poland obtained from the Central Statistics Bureau (Rocznik Statystyczny Głównego Urzedu Statystycznego, 1960; Statystyka ludnosci Głównego Urzedu Statystycznego, 1965). In Table 9 the present results are compared with the corresponding data in England (Gunther and Penrose, 1935) and Denmark (Borberg, 1951).

Table 8

Parental age at birth of affected subjects for (A) sporadic and (B) familial cases in comparison with control age for Poland

	Parents	Mean age in groups studied	Mean age for Poland (control)	Excess over control mean
A	Fathers	32.9±1.97	30.3±0.00667	2.6
	Mothers	28.3±1.88	27.1±0.00874	1.2
B	Fathers	33.3±2.41	30.3±0.00667	3.0
	Mothers	27.2±1.30	27.1±0.00874	0.1

Table 9

Parental age at birth of sporadic cases; Comparison with English and Danish data

Country	Number of cases	Control age fathers	Control age mothers	Excess over control mean fathers	Excess over control mean mothers
England (Gunther and Penrose, 1935)	12	30.9	28.6	0.8	0.3
Denmark (Borberg, 1951)	21	33.3	28.6	0.4	0.5
Poland (1965)	15	30.3	27.1	2.6	1.2

DISCUSSION

We have examined the clinical features of tuberous sclerosis with a view to estimating their diagnostic value and their use in detecting mild and abortive cases, which is of particular importance for achieving as complete ascertainment as possible, an essential prerequisite for a genetical investigation.

Pringle's and Koenen's tumours and shagreen patches are pathognomonic changes, the first being the commonest, present in 36 of 40 subjects in our material. Pedunculated fibromas (mollusca pendula) are less common; café au lait spots are not typical of the disease. Depigmented naevi occurred in 31 instances and their diagnostic importance has been underestimated. Although not pathognomonic, they are especially valuable on account of their high frequency in T.S. and early appearance, being sometimes the earliest visible symptom. Recent reports in the literature confirm their importance (Gold and Freeman, 1965; Crichton, 1966).

Retinal phakomata are also appreciably commoner than usually supposed, being present in almost half of our subjects, as often in mild and abortive as in severely affected examples of the disease. Critchley and Earl found 3 per cent only (1932), Vaas, reviewing the Literature, mentions 8.5 per cent (1940) and others, 25 per cent (Ross and Dickerson, 1943).

Neurological symptoms are common and variable, not pathognomonic for the disease. Severe physical handicap due to damage of the C.N.S. (paralysis, paresis) occurred infrequently (5 per cent). Mental deficiency was found in 28 (70 per cent) of our patients. Estimates by other authors have varied from 34 per cent to 80 per cent (Alliez and Moutin, 1963). Borberg (1951) found 70 per cent. It must be born in mind, however, that methods of ascertainment may usually lead to an overestimate. On the basis of our material affected subjects tend to be severely subnormal or almost normal, intermediate cases being uncommon.

Epilepsy occurred in 33 cases, usually beginning in the first year, most of these in the first six months, A significant feature in our material was spontaneous regression of epilepsy, which died out in seven subjects. This fact is most probably dependent on extinction of activity of the brain foci, and is probably associated with the specific dynamics of the pathological process in T.S. Although observed by others (Schuster, 1914; Critchley and Earl, 1932; Borberg, 1951; Gillis, et al., 1962; Berg and Crome, 1963; MacCarty and Russel, 1958; Kadlubowska, 1959) it has received insufficient attention in the medical literature. It is worth-while noting the frequent occurrence of infantile spasms, which accords with the recent observations of other authors (Gastaut, et al., 1965). This is most probably due to the very early onset of the fits in T.S.

Although one of the three main symptoms of T.S., epilepsy is not pathognomic and its occurrence in a subject alone, does not justify diagnosis, as Pringle's tumours or eye phakomata would. It is common in the general population and might occur by chance in the family of an affected subject.

E.E.G. changes occurred in 20 of 33 subjects examined. Contrary to the views of some other authors (Hartermann, et al., 1957; Hudolin, 1963) it is not of high diagnostic value since changes are infrequent in mild and abortive cases. It seems that there is also a tendency to die out as in epilepsy.

Radiographic appearances may be so specific that diagnosis may be established by them alone. In our material intracranial calcification was seen in 24 subjects and increased density of cranial bones in 26, out of 34 examined. Candle guttering in 16 of 17, internal hydrocephalus in 8 of 17 and cystic changes and cortical thickening of bone in the phalanges of hands in 27 of 33. This is a higher proportion of changes than previously reported, by Holt and Dickerson (1952) for instance, Ross and Dickerson (1943) and others (Berland, 1953). Other, less frequent, findings were tumours and anomalies of the kidneys and renal tracts.

Asymmetry and partial hypertrophy were observed several times. Such changes have also been established in other phakomatoses, such as Von Recklinghausen's disease and Klippel-Trénaunay-Weber's disease.

Genetical Analysis

The incidence of T.S. was estimated by Gunther and Penrose (1935) at 1 in 30,000 in the general population of England and Wales. Ross and Dickerson (1943) estimated an incidence of 0.1 to 0.5 in institutions for mentally retarded epileptics in the U.S.A. Our investigation revealed a 1.1 per cent incidence in similar institutions in Poland and an incidence in the general population of 44×10^{-6}, the highest values so far reported. It seems likely that, as suggested by the clinical observations discussed above, many cases, particularly those with slight expression of skin changes, may often be missed, leading to estimates that are too low. This possibility is supported by the anatomico-pathological studies of Gross and Kattenbeack (1963) who encountered T.S. in 17 of 602 brains of severely subnormal patients.

The mutation rate was estimated by Gunther and Penrose (1935) to be 4 to 8 x 10^{-6}, which is 1 : 120,000 to 1 : 60,000 per person per generation, a figure usually quoted as close to the true frequency. The estimate was based on 20 cases in six of which there was evidence of familial disease, although doubtful in one instance.

Penrose explained abortive T.S. as the consequence of irregular dominance and the action of modifying genes (Penrose, 1934). His first hypothesis assumed three alleles, E the tuberous sclerosis gene, R the normal allele recessive to it, and D an allele dominant to it. The expected proportions of diseased and healthy children from marriages of parents of different genotypes is shown in Table 10. This hypothesis, however, is not born out by our observations, in which the ratio of affected to healthy is 1 : 1, which is not expected on this hypothesis. In Penrose's own data, the ratio was 7 : 5. Moreover, there have been no reports indicating the ED x RR marriage, where both parents would be healthy and disease would be manifest in more than one child.

A later hypothesis of Penrose (Gunther and Penrose, 1935) assumed the modifying gene to be not allelomorphic, and those bearers of a T.S. gene who are homozygous for this allele not manifesting disease, the heterozygotes doing so mildly, the severe form occurring in subjects entirely lacking the modifying gene. By this

94

Table 10

The hypothesis of Penrose (1934) of irregular dominance and the action of modifying genes, assuming a T.S. allele (E) a normal recessive (R) and a normal dominant (D) alleles

	Genotype of parents	Offspring affected	Offspring unaffected
One parent affected	ER × RR	1/2	1/2
	ER × RD	1/4	3/4
	ER × DD	—	1
Both parents unaffected	ED × RR	1/2	1/2
	ED × RD	1/4	3/4
	ED × DD	—	1

hypothesis, if one parent were mildly afflicted, assuming the frequency of the modifying gene to be 1/2 one would expect 5/8 of the children to be healthy, 1/4 to be mildly affected and 1/8 to be severely affected.

Our findings do not accord with these expectations. Almost all affected parents in our material manifested the disease mildly and the ratio of diseased to healthy children was 1 : 1. Later, on the basis of this hypothesis, Penrose estimated the mutation rate at 1 : 40,000 per person per generation, which is 12.5 x 10^{-6} per gene locus per generation (Penrose, 1936). We derived from our data in Poland, an estimate of 11 x 10^{-6} and 14.6 x 10^{-6} if mild mutations leading to familial occurrence of the disease are included.

Genetic Counselling

Of basic importance are : 1. Advice of the risk, to parents with an affected child, of having other affected children; and 2. Advice to mildly affected sibs of an affected subject of their risk of having affected children. In every case a thorough examination of the entire family, including radiography, is essential to determine if the affected subject is the consequence of a fresh mutation or if the condition is familial. If the former, the risk is small, but one cannot be absolutely certain that a case is sporadic.

In cases of high risk the application of contraceptives, induced abortion or sometimes sterilization should be considered.

SUMMARY AND CONCLUSIONS

Clinical

Clinical studies conducted on 40 cases of tuberous sclerosis, besides the well known symptoms of the disease, have revealed the following clinical features which may be useful in the early diagnosis and, what is more, they are quite essential in detection of the abortive cases of the disease.

1. In the group of skin changes, attention is drawn to the frequent appearance of depigmented naevi, second only in frequency to Pringle's tumours, which, considering their early occurrence, form a very important clinical symptom of the disease.

2. Changes in the ocular fundus in the form of retinal nodes appear with much greater frequency (about 50 per cent of the cases) than has commonly been recognised. There was no correlation observed between the intensity of those changes and severity of the disease.

3. Epileptic seizures in tuberous sclerosis in the majority of instances begin to appear in the first year of life often acquiring the form of infantile spasms.

In a considerable proportion of epileptic subjects the phenomenon of "self-cure" of epilepsy is observed.

4. The E.E.G. examination is of less diagnostic value in tuberous sclerosis than usually believed, expecially in the detection of abortive cases. It is probably due to the fact that single foci of cerebral changes display electric activity only within a certain period of time.

5. Radiological changes in the brain, the bones of the skull, and phalanges of hands and feet are very characteristic of tuberous sclerosis and appear with greater frequency than has been indicated so far. They form one of the most valuable diagnostic symptoms of the disease.

Genetical Analysis

1. In cases of familial appearance of the disease dominant inheritance was observed with full penetrance of the tuberous sclerosis gene in spite of varying manifestation. However, it is possible to follow up the disease only in two or three generations which proves a strong selection operating against the gene and resulting in decreased fitness of its carriers.

2. Sporadic cases, probably due to fresh mutations, appear in at least half of the analysed families.

3. The incidence of tuberous sclerosis calculated from this material, which is based on the ascertainment of affected subjects in Poland with severe mental deficiency is about 44×10^{-6}.

4. The mutation rate calculated by a direct method on the basis of the latter data (points 2 and 3) is 11×10^{-6}. Including the mutations leading to mild expression of the disease, which is the condition for appearance of familial cases, the frequency of mutations is probably about 14.6×10^{-6}.

5. The effect of parental age on the incidence of fresh mutations in tuberous sclerosis was not observed to be significant.

ACKNOWLEDGEMENTS

I am grateful to Dr. I. Wald for his help and advice during the whole study, to Dr. Loesch for her assistance in examining many of the patients and for interpreting E.E.G. records, to Dr. P. Kozlowski for interpretation of X-ray pictures, to D. Wójcik for performing psychological assessments in many of the patients and some members of their families, to doctors of the neurological ward of Pruszków's Mental Hospital for their help in clinical examinations, to Dr. A. Kleniewski, Head of the neurological ward in Koszalin for clinical examinations of some of the patients. A special word of gratitude is due to Dr. B. W. Richards for his kind help in writing the extract of the thesis and for correcting the English of the original translation. I am also grateful to Prof. L. S. Penrose for his helpful advice in preparing the present paper.

REFERENCES

ALLIEZ, J. and MOUTIN, P. (1963) L'évolution de l' intelligence chez les sujets atteints de phacomatoses cérébrales. Deuxiéme Colloque International sur les malformations congénitales de l'encéphale - Les phacomatoses cérébrales. *Rev. int. Serv. Santé Armeés.* Numéro hors série, p. 209.

BERG, J. M. and CROME, L. (1963) Les phacomatoses dans la déficience mentale. Deuxième Colloque International sur les malformations congénitales de l' encéphale – les phacomatoses cérébrales. *Rev. int. Serv. Santé Armées.* Numéro hors série, p. 297.

BERLAND, H. I. (1953) Roentgenological findings in tuberous sclerosis : bone manifestation. *Arch. Neurol. Psychiat. (Chic.),* **69**, 669.

BOGAERT, L. VAN (1935) Les dysplasies neuro-ectodermiques congénitales. *Rev. neurol.,* **63**, 353.

BORBERG, A. (1951) *Clinical and genetic investigations into tuberous sclerosis and Recklinghausen's neurofibromatosis.* Opera ex domo biolagiae hereditariae humanae. No. 23 Universitas Hafniensis. *In Acta psychiat. neurol.* Supp. 71.

BOURNEVILLE (1880) Contribution à l'étude de l'idiotie (obs. III : Sclérose tubéreuse des circonvolutions cérébrales; idiotie et épilepsie hémiplégique). *Arch. Neurol. (Paris),* **1**, 69.

CORNEE, J. and LE BRAS, M. (1964) Sclérose tubéreuse de Bourneville. Premier cas africain. *Méd. trop.,* **24**, 470.

CRICHTON, J. U. (1966) Infantile spasms and skin anomalies. *Develop. Med. Child Neurol.,* **8**, 273.

CRITCHLEY, M. and EARL, C. J. C. (1932) Tuberose sclerosis and allied conditions. *Brain,* **55**, 311.

GASTAUT, H., ROGER, J., SOULAYROL, R., SALAMON, G., REGIS, H. and LOB, H. (1965) Encephalopathie myoclonique infantile avec hypsarythmie (syndrome de West) et sclérose tubéreuse de Bourneville. *J. Neurol. Sci.,* **2**, 140

GILLIS, E., RONSE, H. and ANDRE-BALISAUX, G. (1962) A propos d'un cas d'épiloïa : quelques considérations sur les geno-neuro-dermatoses. *Arch. Belg. Derm. Syph.,* **18**, 161.

GOLD, A. P. and FREEMAN, J. M. (1965) Depigmented nevi : the earliest sign of tuberous sclerosis. *Pediatrics,* **35**, 1003.

GREBE, H. (1955) *Chondrodysplasia.* Roma : Istituto Gregorio Mendel.

GROSS, H. and KATTENBEACK, E. (1963) La mégalencéphalie et sa position au sein de phacomatoses. Deuxième Colloque International sur les malformations congénitales de l'encéphale. Les phacomatoses cérébrales. *Rev. int. Serv. Santé Armées. Numéro hors série,* p. 521.

GUNTHER, M. and PENROSE, L. S. (1935) The genetics of epiloia. *J. Genet.,* **31**, 413.

HARTERMANN, P., DUREUX, J. B. and MARTIN, J. (1957) Considérations ophtalmologiques et électroencéphalographiques sur 31 observations de sclérose tubéreuse de Bourneville et de neurofibromatose de Recklinghausen. *Rev. Oto-neuro-ophtal.,* **29**, 216.

HERMANS, E. H., GROSFELD, J. C. M. and SPAAS, J. A. J. (1965) The fifth phacomatosis. *Dermatologica (Basel)*, **130**, 446.

HOEVE, J. VAN DER (1923) Eye diseases in tuberose sclerosis of the brain and in Recklinghausen's disease. *Trans. Ophthal. Soc. U.U.*, **43**, 534.

HOLT, J. F. and DICKERSON, W. W. (1952) The osseous lesions of tuberous sclerosis. *Radiology*, **58**, 1.

HUDOLIN, V. (1963) Tuberozna skleroza. *Anali Bolnice "Dr. M. Stojanowic"*, *2, supl.* **5**, 92.

KADLUBOWSKA, K. (1959) Przypadek choroby Bourneville'a (sclerosis tuberosa cerebri.) *Klin. oczna*, **29**, 395.

LOESCH, D., ZAREMBA, J., KOLACKA, M. and DYMECKI, J. (1966) W sprawie zwiazku nerwowo-skórnej melanoblastozy (Touraine) z fakomatozami. *Neurol. Neurochir. Psychiat. pol.*, **16**, 265.

MacCARTY, W. C. and RUSSELL, D. G. (1958) Tuberous sclerosis; report of a case with ependymoma. *Radiology*, **71**, 833.

PENROSE, L. S. (1934) *The influence of heredity on disease*. London: H. K. Lewis.

PENROSE, L. S. (1936) Autosomal mutation and modification in man with special reference to mental defect. *Ann. Eugen. (Lond.)*, **7**, 1.

PENROSE, L. S. (1956) Mutation in man. *Acta genet. (Basel)*, **6**, 169.

RANDAZZO, S. D. and GREPPI, P. (1964) Contributo allo studio della malattia di Bourneville-Pringle. A proposito di un caso associato a neurofibromatosi di Recklinghausen. *Minerva derm.*, **39**, 316.

ROSS, A. T. and DICKERSON, W. W. (1943) Tuberous sclerosis. *Arch. Neurol. Psychiat. (Chic.)*, **50**, 233.

SCHUSTER, P. (1913) Beiträge zur Klinik der tuberösen Sklerose des Gehirns. *Dtsch. Z. Nervenheilk.*, **50**, 96.

SHERLOCK, E. B. (1911) *The feeble-minded*. London: MacMillan.

SHINFUKU, N. and KADOWSKI, T. (1962) Clinical studies on 10 cases of sclerosis tuberosa. *J. Yonago med. Ass.*, **13**, 216.

TOURAINE, A. (1955) *L'hérédité en médecine*. Paris: Mason.

UNTERHARNSCHEIDT, F. (1964) Uber einen disontogenetischen Prozess mit blastomatösem Einschlag (tuberöse Sklerose) beim Affen. *Acta Neuropath. (Berl.)*, **3**, 250.

VAAS, J. (1940) Klinik und Erbgang der tuberösen Sklerose. *Arch. Psychiat. Nervenkr.*, **111**, 547.

WAARDENBURG, P. J., FRANCESCHETTI, A., KLEIN, D. (1963) *Genetics and ophtalmology*. Assen: Royal Van Gorcum Ltd. Vol. 2, p. 109.

WALD, I. and STOMMA, D. (1965) Epidemiologia glebokiego uposledzenia umyslowego w Polsce. *Sympozjum Psychiatrii Dzieciecej, Szczecin. Proceedings, Gdansk,* 145.

WEINBERG, W. (1912) Ueber Methode und Fehlerquellen der Untersuchung auf Mendelsche Zahlen beim Menschen. *Arch. Rass.-u. GesBiol.*, **9**, 165.

YAKOVLEV, P. I. and GUTHRIE, R. H. (1931) Congenital ectodermoses (neurocutaneous syndromes) in epileptic patients. *Arch. Neurol. Psychiat. (Chic.)*, **26**, 1145.

98

CYSTATHIONINURIA AND

RENAL IMINOGLYCINURIA IN A PEDIGREE

A Perspective on Counseling

DONALD T. WHELAN, M.D., AND CHARLES R. SCRIVER, M.D.

Abstract Cystathioninuria and hyperglycinuria both occurred in a male Ashkenazi-Jewish infant. Both traits were dominantly inherited as the heterozygous forms of two independent mutant alleles. The patient was thus a double heterozygote. Renal iminoglycinuria appeared as an autosomal recessive trait in the mother of the proband and in four of her sibs. This condition is the homozygous form of the trait that presents as hyperglycinuria in the heterozygote; it is a benign inborn error of amino acid transport. Cystathioninuria is probably also a benign trait. Knowledge of the precise phenotypes and their significance were of practical value in counseling the family.

HARRIS and colleagues[1] reported the first case of cystathioninuria. Since then five additional patients, presumably homozygous for the hereditary trait, have been described in the literature,[2-6] and at least three others are known to exist.[7,8] The problem of cystathioninuria and the relevant aspects of vitamin B_6 metabolism were reviewed, and some of the original case studies brought up to date in the recent Symposium on Treatment of Amino Acid Disorders.[9] We have investigated a male infant with persistent cystathioninuria who was at first thought to be homozygous for the inherited form of the trait. Subsequent studies revealed that he was actually a heterozygote, and that the striking initial cystathioninuria probably reflected a transient hepatic disturbance. The propositus also had persistent hyperglycinuria; investigation of this led to the discovery of a second inherited hyperaminoaciduria — namely, renal iminoglycinuria in the same family. The appearance of two inborn errors of amino acid metabolism in a single family without known consanguinity is most unusual. This paper describes such a case, and illustrates how knowledge of the precise phenotype in the propositus, gained through a simple exercise in biochemical genetics, helped us counsel the family and care for the patient.

CASE REPORT

D.S., the propositus for the pedigree (Fig. 1), an Ashkenazi-Jewish infant, became jaundiced at 4 days of age, apparently because of a urinary-tract infection. The highest recorded value for total bilirubin in plasma was 11.5 mg per 100 ml, of which 6.4 mg was conjugated. The highest recorded values for other tests of liver function were found in the 2d week of life, and were as follows: serum glutamic oxalacetic transaminase, 130 units; glutamic pyruvic transaminase, 66 units; alkaline phosphatase, 45 King–Armstrong units; and cholesterol, 140 mg per 100 ml. Under antibiotic treatment, the jaundice disappeared by the 6th week after birth. Examination of the amino acids in urine by 2-dimensional partition chromatography on filter paper[10] during the 5th week of life revealed an unusual large ninhydrin-positive spot in the region of phosphoethanolamine and cystathionine; the substance was subsequently proved to be cystathionine. The patient was lost to follow-up observation until he was 5 months old. His growth and development were normal in the interim, and he was considered to be healthy. He received a normal diet, which could not be considered deficient in vitamin B_6. On admission to The Montreal Children's Hospital, the infant appeared to be well nourished and normally proportioned. The measurements of head circumference, weight and height each fell on the 25th percentile. In particular, the liver was normally palpable at the right costal margin.

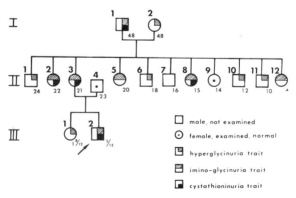

FIGURE 1. Pedigree Containing Three Traits: Cystathioninuria; Hyperglycinuria; and Iminoglycinuria.

Urinalysis was within normal limits. The total plasma protein was 7.2 gm, the blood urea nitrogen 26 mg, and the bilirubin, 0.4 mg total and 0.2 mg direct per 100 ml. The fasting blood sugar was 79 mg per 100 ml. The serum glutamic oxalacetic transaminase was 42 units, and the glutamic pyruvic transaminase 26 units. Prothrombin time, plasma alkaline phosphatase, cephalin flocculation and thymol turbidity, were all normal. The hemoglobin was 10.5 gm per 100 ml. The mean corpuscular hemoglobin concentration was 34 per cent and the reticulocytes 0.5 per cent. The platelet count was 625,000, and the white-cell count 9700, with normal differential. The urinary catecholamine excretion rate in timed urine collections was normal on 3 occasions.

The family history disclosed that the maternal grandparents of the propositus are healthy Ashkenazi-Jews, who emigrated from London, England, to Canada in 1947. There are 11 clinically healthy children from their marriage; no miscarriages or prenatal deaths occurred. The mother of the propositus had 1 previous normal pregnancy. There is no identified consanguinity in the pedigree.

SPECIAL INVESTIGATIONS

Cystathioninuria

The identity of cystathionine in the urine of the propositus was confirmed by several procedures. The ninhydrin-positive compound in urine cochromatographed with a sample of pure L-cystathionine in seven chromatographic systems, as follows: one-dimensional partition chromatography on filter paper in three solvent systems consisting of butanol, acetic acid and water (12:3:5), phenol and water, and 2,6-lutidine and water (2.2:1); two-dimensional chromatography with the phenol-lutidine combination; high-voltage electrophoresis on filter paper, followed by partition chromatography[11]; and regular and modified[12] elution chromatography on ion-exchange resin, with the use of a Beckman–Spinco semiautomatic amino acid analyzer.

The endogenous renal clearance of cystathionine, calculated on a three-hour urine collection, was 147 ml per minute per $1.73M^2$ when the concentration in plasma was 0.001 mM (0.022 mg per 100 ml). Although this concentration in plasma is abnormally high (normal is "zero"[4]), it is still only about one twentieth of the value observed in those who are homozygous for the trait.[2,4,9] A prerenal origin for the cystathioninuria in this patient and the anticipated high endogenous renal clearance of this amino acid[2,13] are both evident from these data.

Following a load of L-methionine (100 mg per kilogram of body weight) by mouth the concentration of methionine in plasma rose to 0.9 mM (13.4 mg per 100 ml) and then returned to normal within 24 hours (Fig. 2). This is the normal response.[14] The amount of cystathionine in plasma increased after the methionine load, and cystathionine excretion in the urine also rose abnormally.[14] A similar response has been observed in homozygous patients, but in those cases the accumulation of cystathionine was greater. Administration of pyridoxine to homozygotes alters the response to methionine loading,[2,4-6,9] so that it resembles the response described in our untreated propositus.

After a load of L-tryptophan (100 mg per kilogram) by mouth there was no significant increase in the excretion of xanthurenic acid; this and other tryptophan metabolites were analyzed by two-dimensional paper chromatography by the methods of Jepson.[15] These negative results indicate that vitamin B_6 deficiency was not the cause for the abnormal excretion of cystathionine in this patient.[9,16,17] Cystathionine excretion was suppressed to normal values after the daily administration of pyridoxine (Fig. 2).

Cystathionine excretion in urine was measured in fasting morning urine samples in all available members of the immediate family by elution chromatography on ion-exchange resin. An obvious cystathio-

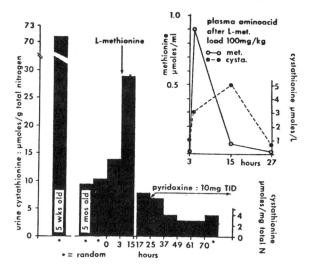

FIGURE 2. *Response of Urinary and Plasma Cystathionine to Methionine Loading and Pyridoxine in the Propositus.*

nine peak was seen on the elution chromatograms in four subjects other than the propositus (Fig. 1). Dominant inheritance of the trait is seen in this pedigree. The excretion of cystathionine by the mother and the paternal grandfather was equivalent to that of the propositus (Table 1).

Iminoglycinuria

Urinary excretion of glycine by the propositus was unusually high (Table 1). The concentration of glycine in plasma was normal, and the endogenous renal clearance of this amino acid was elevated (20.8 ml per minute per 1.73M^2 whereas the normal value is less than 8.6 ml).[18] The renal clearance of other amino acids (except cystathionine) was normal.

The hyperglycinuric trait was apparently inherited from the mother, who exhibited an iminoglycinuric phenotype (Table 1 and Fig. 1). Both maternal grandparents were hyperglycinuric; their other children exhibited a phenotype that was either iminoglycinuric or hyperglycinuric or normal. The pattern of inheritance of the iminoglycinuria trait is clearly shown in this pedigree and has been confirmed in two others.[19] The hyperglycinuric trait is inherited dominantly and resembles the trait described by deVries et al.[20] The iminoglycinuric trait is a recessive phenotype. The former trait thus represents the heterozygous, and the latter the homozygous, form of a mutation involving a pair of alleles at the gene locus that specifies a tubular transport system common to the imino acids and glycine.[21,22] The detailed investigation of this inborn error of amino acid transport in this and two other pedigrees is the subject of other communications.[19,23]

The propositus has thus demonstrated inherited traits for mutant alleles that are at different loci and control independent aspects of amino acid metabolism. The infant is therefore a double heterozygote for two rare inborn errors. The data available on this pedigree indicate that close linkage between the two sets of alleles is most unlikely.

DISCUSSION

Our interest in the propositus came by chance when urine was sent for chromatographic screening to help with the clinical management. Cystathionine is not seen on the chromatogram of urinary amino

103

TABLE 1. *Urinary Excretion of Relevant Amino Acids in Family Members.*

SUBJECT	TRAIT* EXPRESSED & PRESUMED GENOTYPE†	CYSTATHIONINE		GLYCINE	PROLINE	HYDROXYPROLINE
		μmole/gm of total nitrogen	mg/gm of creatinine	μmole/gm of total nitrogen	μmole/gm of total nitrogen	μmole/gm of total nitrogen
III, 2 (propositus)	C(het), G (het)	71‡	343	343	0	0
I, 1	C(het), G (het)	9.7-14§	91-142	260-600	0	0
I, 2	G (het)	4	20	283	0	0
II, 1	G (het)	4	8	549	0	0
II, 2	C(het), IG(hom)	5	10	182	7	–
II, 3 (mother)	C(het), IG(hom)	13	23	1,055	233	40
II, 4 (father)	Normal	0		1,276	0	0
II, 5	IG(hom)	1		1,439	34	30
II, 6	G (het)	1		172	0	0
II, 8	C(het), IG(hom)	7	16	496	241	94
II, 9	Normal	2		114	0	0
II, 10	G (het)	0		437	0	0
II, 11	G (het)	0.5		305	0	0
II, 12	IG(hom)	0		307	53	22
III, 1	G (het)	1	6	200	0	0
Normal value		Trace (<4.5)¶	Trace (<10)	<160**	0**	0**

*C = cystathioninuria; G = hyperglycinuria; IG = iminoglycinuria.

†Het = heterozygote; Hom = homozygote.

‡1st sample, at 5 wk of age.

§On readmission at 5 mo of age.

¶Derived from Brenton et al[11] & Scriver & Davies.[14]

||Arbitrary value, based on literature on cystathioninuria.[13]

**Scriver & Davies[14] & Scriver.[15]

acids from normal persons. The cause of the marked cystathioninuria in this patient was at first not clear. It seemed evident that cystathioninuria secondary to neuroblastoma[24] could be eliminated. A hepatic disturbance,[25] although perhaps of some significance on the first examination at five weeks of age, could also be eliminated as a cause of the persistent cystathioninuria. Clinical and biochemical evidence also ruled against vitamin B_6 deficiency as a cause for the cystathioninuria.[9,16,17] It was concluded that the origin of the condition (trait) was hereditary. We were impressed by the amount of cystathioninuria present in the first sample sent to us; because we had no prior experience with the condition, and were under pressure because of the impending departure of the patient for Israel (scheduled to occur four days after the readmission), we decided to treat the patient with pyridoxine as if he were a homozygote. When the investigation of the pedigree was completed, and when our data were compared with those in the literature, it became obvious that the trait in the propositus reflected not the homozygous, but the heterozygous, phenotype. Since untreated cystathioninuric heterozygotes are otherwise normal, there is no reason to administer pyridoxine for therapeutic purposes; the Israeli physicians to whom the patient was referred were therefore informed that the pyridoxine medication could be discontinued. One might question in passing whether pyridoxine treatment is even indicated for homozygotes. No consistent clinical phenotype has been identified with the biochemical trait, and some subjects are known to be healthy.[7] Therefore, one wonders whether the cystathioninuric trait is actually harmful. If this point is not defined, against what clinical criteria can one judge the assumed clinical efficacy of pyridoxine therapy?

The rare cystathioninuria trait is particularly interesting because of its frequent occurrence with other known hereditary diseases. Phenylketonuria[3,9] has been found in one patient, and nephrogenic diabetes insipidus[6] in another propositus with cystathioninuria. The present case is the third of concurrence of cystathioninuria and a second hereditary trait in a propositus. The significance of this tendency for hereditary cystathioninuria to occur in conjunction with other diseases is unknown, but should not be ignored, particularly in view of the unusual

105

mechanism proposed for the primary abnormality of cystathionine metabolism (as indicated in papers by Frimpter and Scriver[9]).

The second hereditary trait (hyperglycinuria) observed in the propositus is widespread, and one observed in many forms.[26] We have recently discerned[19,23] that the particular type of hyperglycinuria described here represents the heterozygous form of an autosomal recessive trait, whose fully expressed phenotype is iminoglycinuria. The iminoglycinuria mutation (or mutations) are harmless to the best of our knowledge, and this information helped us further in counseling this family. The excretion of proline, hydroxyproline and glycine in urine is a normal trait in all newborn human infants. The persistence of the trait represents a hereditary disorder of amino acid transport analogous to conditions such as classic cystinuria and Hartnup disease.[27] In the iminoglycinuric phenotype, a cellular transport system common to proline and hydroxyproline and glycine is affected. There is some evidence that more than one allele at a single gene locus controls this transport system.[19] The concept is analogous to Rosenberg's[28] interpretation of the genetic control of the dibasic transport system for which at least three alleles at a single locus are proposed.

We are indebted to Miss Eluned Davies, Mrs. Carol Clow, Mr. Peter Lamm and Dr. L. Linarelli, for technical assistance and to Dr. Oscar Singer, who kindly referred the patient.

REFERENCES

1. Harris, H., Penrose, L. S., and Thomas, D. H. H. Cystathioninuria. *Ann. Human Genet.* **23**:442-453, 1959.
2. Frimpter, G. W., Haymovitz, A., and Horwith, M. Cystathioninuria. *New Eng. J. Med.* **268**:333-339, 1963.
3. Shaw, K. N. F., et al. Cystathioninuria in phenylketonuric patient. Presented at meeting of Society for Pediatric Research, Atlantic City, New Jersey, May 1 and 2, 1963.
4. Berlow, S. Studies in cystathioninemia. *Am. J. Dis. Child.* **112**:135-142, 1966.
5. Mongeau, J.-G., Hilgartner, M., Worthen, H. G., and Frimpter, G. W. Cystathioninuria: study of infant with normal mentality, thrombocytopenia, and renal calculi. *J. Pediat.* **69**:1113-1120, 1966.
6. Perry, T. L., Robinson, G. C., Teasdale, J. M., and Hansen, S. Concurrence of cystathioninuria, nephrogenic diabetes insipidus and severe anemia. *New Eng. J. Med.* **276**:721-725, 1967.
7. Hardwick, D. Personal communication.
8. Szeinberg, A. Personal communication.
9. Symposium: treatment of amino acid disorders. *Am. J. Dis. Child.* **113**:1-174, 1967.

10. Dent, C. E. Study of behaviour of some sixty amino-acids and other ninhydrin-reacting substances on phenol-'collidine' filter-paper chromatograms, with notes as to occurrence of some of them in biological fluids. *Biochem. J.* **43**:169-180, 1948.

11. Efron, M. L. Two-way separation of amino acids and other ninhydrin-reacting substances by high-voltage electrophoresis followed by paper chromatography. *Biochem. J.* **72**:691-694, 1959.

12. Scriver, C. R., Davies, E., and Lamm, P. Accelerated selective short column chromatography of neutral and acidic amino acids on Beckman-Spinco analyzer, modified for simultaneous analysis of two samples. *Clin. Biochem.* **1**:179-191, 1968.

13. Frimpter, G. W., and Greenberg, A. J. Renal clearance of cystathionine in homozygous and heterozygous cystathioninuria, cystinuria and normal state. *J. Clin. Investigation* **46**:975-982, 1967.

14. Brenton, D. P., Cusworth, D. C., and Gaull, G. E. Homocystinuria: metabolic studies on 3 patients. *J. Pediat.* **67**:58-68, 1965.

15. Jepson, J. B. Indoles and related Ehrlich reactors. In *Chromatographic and Electrophoretic Techniques.* Second edition. Edited by I. Smith. 2 vol. Vol. I. *Chromatography.* New York: Interscience, 1961.

16. Scriver, C. R., and Hutchison, J. H. Vitamin B_6 deficiency syndrome in human infancy: biochemical and clinical observations. *Pediatrics* **31**:240-250, 1963.

17. Fourman, P., Summerscales, J. W., and Morgan, D. M. Cystathioninuria from pyridoxine deficiency complicating treatment of hypercalcaemia in cretin. *Arch. Dis. Childhood* **41**:273-278, 1966.

18. Scriver, C. R., and Davies, E. Endogenous renal clearance rates of free amino acids in pre-pubertal children: employing accelerated procedure for elution chromatography of basic amino acids on ion exchange resin. *Pediatrics* **36**:592-598, 1965.

19. Scriver, C. R. Renal tubular transport of proline, hydroxyproline and glycine. III. Genetic basis for more than one mode of uptake in human kidney. *J. Clin. Investigation* (in press).

20. Vries, A. de, Kochwa, S., Lazebnik, J., Frank, M., and Djaldetti, M. Glycinuria, hereditary disorder associated with nephrolithiasis. *Am. J. Med.* **23**:408-415, 1957.

21. Scriver, C. R., and Goldman, H. Renal tubular transport of proline, hydroxyproline, and glycine. II. Hydroxy-l-proline as substrate and as inhibitor in vivo. *J. Clin. Investigation* **45**:1357-1363, 1966.

22. Scriver, C. R., Efron, M. L., and Schafer, I. A. Renal tubular transport of proline, hydroxyproline, and glycine in health and in familial hyperprolinemia. *J. Clin. Investigation* **43**:374-385, 1964.

23. Scriver, C. R., and Wilson, O. H. Amino acid transport: evidence for genetic control of two types in human kidney. *Science* **155**:1428-1430, 1967.

24. Gjessing, L. R. Studies of functional neural tumors. II. Cystathioninuria. *Scandinav. J. Clin. & Lab. Investigation* **15**:474-478, 1963.

25. Lieberman, E., Shaw, K. N. F., and Donnell, G. N. Cystathioninuria in galactosemia and certain types of liver disease. *Pediatrics* **40**:828-833, 1967.

26. Wyngaarden, J. B., and Segal, S. Hyperglycinurias. In *The Metabolic Basis of Inherited Disease.* Second edition. Edited by J. B. Stanbury, J. B. Wyngaarden and D. S. Fredrickson. New York: McGraw-Hill, 1966. Pp. 341-352.

27. Milne, M. D. Disorders of amino-acid transport. *Brit. M. J.* **1**:327-336, 1964.

28. Rosenberg, L. E. Cystinuria: genetic heterogeneity and allelism. *Science* **154**:1341-1343, 1966.

Supported in part by grants from the Medical Research Council of Canada (MT-1085), the National Institutes of Health, United States Public Health Service (AM-05117) and the Department of National Health and Welfare, Canada (604-7-459).

Genetic Counselling in Lobster-Claw Anomaly:

Discussion of Variability of Genetic Influence in Different Families

MIECZYLAWA JAWORSKA, M.D., DR. JERZY POPIOLEK

Several problems are inherent in genetic counselling with regard to the interesting hereditary malformation of cleft hand and foot, the so-called lobster-claw deformity. This anomaly, a disturbance in development of the central ray of the embryonic hand and foot, results in the absence or extreme hypoplasia of corresponding phalanges and of central metatarsal or metacarpal bones; there is also a soft tissue disorder leading to fusion of the medial and lateral digits into two masses. A deep cleft separates the affected palm into the ulnar and radial components, or the foot into the tibial and fibular components. These curve against each other, giving the appearance of pincers of a lobster.[1]

The abnormal genetic influence exerts its teratogenic effect about the seventh week of embryonic life, affecting the differentiation of hand and foot plates. Since the tendency to bone formation remains unaffected, however, secondary displacement of bones and fusion of bones take place. In all cases reported to date, when the hands were affected there were foot defects as well. The variability of the deformities is greater, however, in the hands than in the feet.[6]

Case Descriptions

Case 1. J. K., a 12-month-old boy, was the first child born to his parents. Pregnancy and labor were normal. Neither parent had congenital malformations, and both were in good health. There was no family history of congenital anomalies.

Clinical Description (Fig. 1)

Hands: The palm is divided into lateral and medial radiants which are turned towards each other. The cleft between the metacarpals is complete.

Feet: In each foot two digits are missing. The nails of both great toes are deformed. The third and fourth digits of the right foot are partially fused and curved at a 60° angle. Deep cleavage is present up to the metatarsals. The left foot is less typical, the central ray being represented by hypoplastic middle toe.

Case 2. T. J. is also a 12-month-old boy whose mother experienced a threatened abortion during the early weeks of gestation and of heavy emotional shock secondary to her husband's arrest and imprisonment. Three previous pregnancies had resulted in spontaneous abortions, and another one in miscarriage. The patient is the only living child.

The child has a lobster-claw anomaly plus a complete cleft of his primary palate and an inguinal hernia (Fig. 2). His grandfather's sister had a son with a similar anomaly of his hands and feet (Fig. 3).

Clinical Description

Hands: The second and third fingers of the right hand are missing. The cleft of this hand separates the palm into two parts, and the distal phalanx of the thumb is curved medially at a 90° angle. The left hand is normal except for mild brachydactyly.

Feet: On both feet, the second toe as well as the distal phalanx of the fourth and fifth toes are missing. A mild central cleft is present.

109

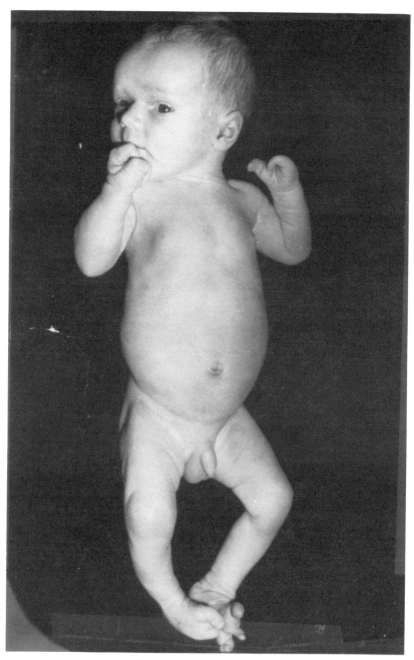

FIG. 1. Case 1. Twelve-month-
old boy with lobster-claw anomaly of hands and feet. Family
history is negative for similar
congenital defects.

110

Case 3. L. J. is a 19-year-old boy with lobster-claw anomaly. Figure 4 is a pedigree of the paternal line. It shows the finding of this same defect among five of seven males and one of seven females in the family. Figure 5 shows the patient, his father and his 14-year-old brother, and Figure 6 is a photo of their hands and feet. Their deformed feet are presented in Figures 7–9 in order to demonstrate their surprising similarity. Figure 10 is a picture and Figure 11 is a radiogram of the patient's hands.

The pattern of inheritance in this family strongly suggests transmission of the lobster-claw trait as an autosomal dominant gene with complete penetrance. Evidence for this is its transmission through four successive generations in the paternal line. There were no consanguineous marriages detected in this family.

The regular expressivity of this gene is manifest in the identically malformed feet. The patient's hands do show some deviation from the pattern observed in two other relatives. This is most likely the result of greater variation in secondary distortion of bone and soft tissue elements.

Clinical Description

The patient's anomaly (Figs. 8, 10, 11) shows all the typical features of lobster-claw anomaly: the clefts, absence of digits, syndactyly either by bone or soft tissues, a tendency to overgrowth of digits, and the presence of cross bones. The hands and feet were bilaterally symmetrical in every detail.

Discussion of Problems in
Genetic Counselling

Our cases contribute to the total picture of the genetic problem of claw hand and foot anomalies. They illustrate also that the genetic prognosis is not always uniform.

In the third family, high penetration and a regular expressivity of a dominant gene sufficiently establishes a high risk for future offspring. The reverse is true in the second family. Here, low gene penetration enables us to be more optimistic. In this case too, there may be some modifying factor involved in the genetic background responsible for a low incidence of anomaly and the high rate of phenotypically normal individuals. It may be

111

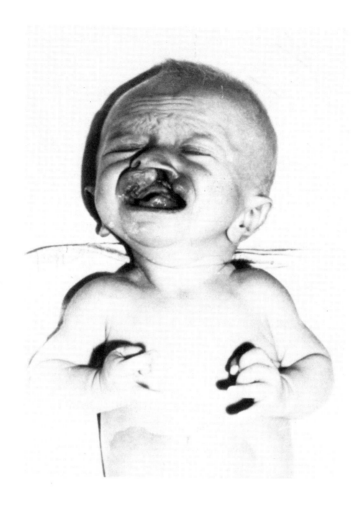

Fig. 2. Case 2. Twelve-month-old boy with lobster-claw anomaly plus complete cleft of his primary palate and an inguinal hernia.

concluded that the "own" specific genotype of a particular family is largely responsible for the regularity of genetic manifestation.

Complications of the mother's pregnancy in Case 2 are unlikely to be a chance association. It is well known that environmental factors acting on the fetus which is genetically predisposed to anomaly, increase the risk of malformation.

112

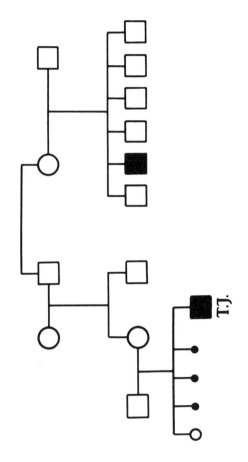

FIG. 3. The pedigree of Case 2 is pictured showing low gene penetrance.

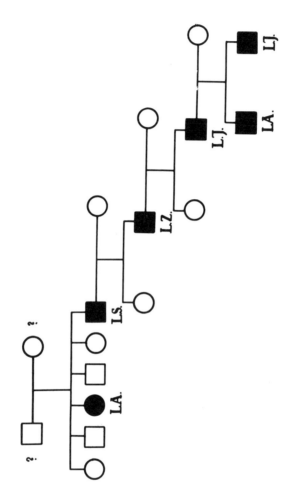

FIG. 4. The pedigree of Case 3 showing five boys and one girl affected. The patient is L. J.

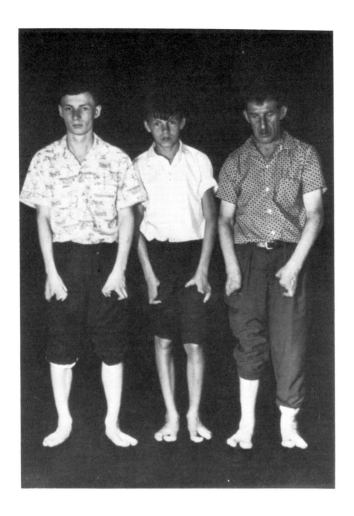

FIG. 5. Father and his two sons described under Case 3 are shown. All have lobster-claw anomaly.

Genetic counseling in Case 1 is the most difficult. We cannot reliably tell the parents of this child whether or not the child's malformation is hereditary in their family. A fresh mutation is a distinct possibility and occasionally this mutation may occur so early in the parental germ cell line that more than one sibling is affected in the first generation.[3] One author notes that bilaterally symmetrical defects are likely to be mutations; unilateral

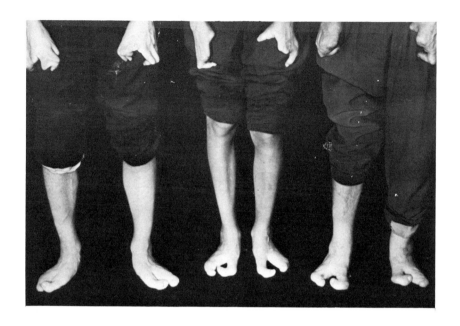

FIG. 6. Close up of the hands and feet of the father
and two sons in Case 3.

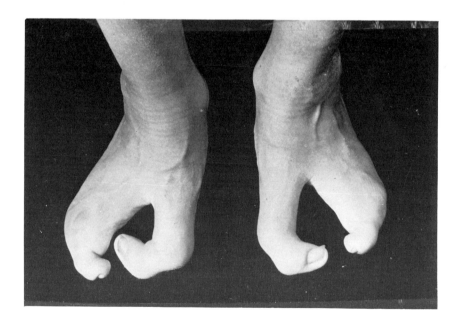

FIG. 7. The feet of the father in Figure 8 are shown.
Note marked similarity to Figure 9.

116

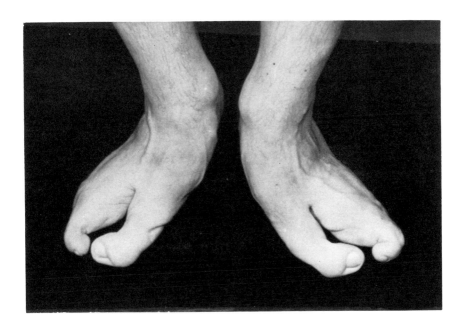

FIG. 8. The feet of the patient (Case 3) are shown.

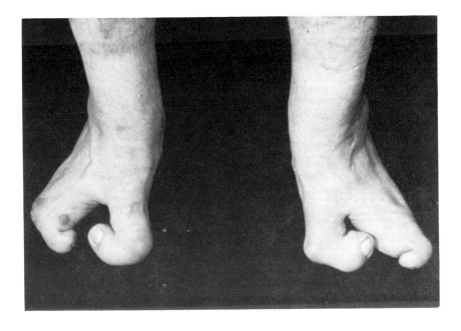

FIG. 9. The feet of Case 3's younger brother are shown.

117

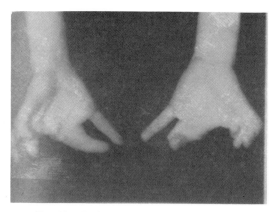

FIG. 10. The hands of Case 3 are pictured.

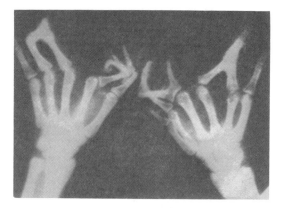

FIG. 11. Roentgenogram of the hands of Case 3 showing bony bridging and other marked development abnormalities.

defects or those limited to one limb are usually due to environmental teratogenic agents.

Even if we accept the premise that a fresh mutation was responsible for the apparently sporadic anomaly in Case 1, it is still impossible to predict the fate of this and the next generation. Gene penetrance may either follow the pattern observed in the other two families described above, or the gene expression may not be so regular. In this event, the deformity might be variably manifest in certain relatives in any degree of severity from webbing of the fingers to the extreme lobster-claw form.[5]

The predominant incidence among boys in the family of Case 3 agrees with Walker's[8] series where the ratio is 20 males to 16 females and with Myer's[4] in which boys outnumber girls 11 to one. Rao[7] also reports seven individuals affected in one family, all of them males. The over-all ratio of 43 boys to 18 girls (our cases included) even encompasses that expected if an inherited trait is lethal in the female. The ability of this gene to be lethal, yet only cause an anomaly which does not interfere with survival and longevity, seems very unlikely.

The defect is probably merely sex-limited, with only occasional expression in the female. To account further for the predominance in boys, it should also be pointed out that the hand bones among females develop earlier in embryonic life than the corresponding bones in males. Since the gene produces its teratogenic effect at about seven weeks gestation, the differentiation of the hand and foot plates in the female embryo has already advanced according to the normal plan of development, and the effect of the gene may, thus, not be manifest in girls.

Whatever is the true interpretation, however, the risk to males of having the lobster-claw anomaly is far greater than for females, regardless of any variable manifestation of the gene in particular families.

Lobster-claw anomaly usually represents an isolated defect. A variety of associated malformations have been reported, but appear to be infrequent and irregular. The association with cleft of primary palate deserves special attention, since facial clefts are known to be frequently associated with deformities of the limbs. One author[8] reports three cases of lobster-claw anomaly associated with cleft of both the primary and secondary palate.

119

REFERENCES

1. Barsky, A.J., "Cleft Hand: Classification, Incidence and Treatment," *Journal of Bone and Joint Surgery*, 1964, 46-A:1707.

2. Bunnel, S., "Surgery of the Hand," *J.B. Lippincott Co.*, Philadelphia, Montreal, part 4, 1948, 793.

3. Fraser, F.C., "Recent Advances in Genetics in Relation to Pediatrics," *Journal of Pediatrics*, 1958, 52:734.

4. Mayer — cited by Walker /8/

5. Montagu, F., "A Pedigree of Syndactylism of the Middle and Ring Fingers," *American Journal of Human Genetics*, 1953, 5:356.

6. Moyson, F., "Les Malformations des Membres," Bruxelles-med., 1963, 43:735.

7. Rao, Y.G., "Split Foot and Split Hand," *Indian Journal of Medical Science*, 1963, 17:352.

8. Walker, J.C.; and L. Clodius, "The Syndrome of Cleft Lip, Cleft Palate and Lobster-Claw Deformities of the Hands and Feet," *Plastic and Reconstructive Surgery*, 1963, 32:627.

Risk to Offspring of Parents With Congenital Heart Defects

James J. Nora, MD; Paul F. Dodd, MD; Dan G. McNamara, MD; Michael A. W. Hattwick, MD; Robert D. Leachman, MD; and Denton A. Cooley, MD

The occurrence risk of atrial-septal defect (ASD) and ventricular-septal defect (VSD) was determined in children of 308 adults with these heart lesions, most of which had been surgically corrected. Parents with ASD had 2.6% of their children affected with ASD which is 37 times greater than the estimated population frequency. For VSD, 3.7% of the children of parents with this heart defect were similarly affected. This is 21 times the estimated population frequency. These findings are offered as empirical risk figures for the purposes of genetic counseling. The data were found to approximate closely the predictions of multifactorial inheritance hypothesis for the etiology of congenital heart diseases. In comparing the congenital heart patients with the general population, differences in marriage patterns were detected which could influence fertility and partially offset the increased recurrence risk.

THE WIDESPREAD employment and excellent therapeutic results of surgical correction of congenital cardiovascular defects have introduced a problem that requires an answer. There are many patients with congenital cardiac malformations who are reaching reproductive age and who would not have survived had it not been for recent advances in medical and surgical management of those lesions. These patients want to know what the chances are that their children may also have congenital heart defects. A corollary question that society may wish to ask is: Are we to expect an increasing incidence of congenital heart diseases as the result of recent therapeutic advances?

The following study was performed to determine the prevalence of congenital cardiac anomalies among the children of adults who have had ventricular-septal defect (VSD) or atrial-septal defect (ASD), and are now in the reproductive age range. The patients also provided an opportunity to test the multifactorial inheritance hypothesis for the etiology of congenital heart diseases.

Clinical Material and Methods

The index cases for this investigation were 308 adults with VSD or ASD confirmed by cardiac catheterization. Of these patients, 262 were postoperative. The lower limits of age for admission to the study was 21 years for women and 25 years for men.

Contact was made during hospitalization, at outpatient visits, or by mailed questionnaire. All children of the index cases who could reasonably be examined by the investigators were so examined. Reports of local physicians were also employed. However, all cases diagnosed as congenital heart lesions were personally evaluated by the investigators by physical examination, electrocardiographic and roentgenographic studies, or by referring to autopsy records.

Results

Table 1 shows the characteristics of the population sampled, the preponderance of women with ASD, and the approximate equality between the sexes with VSD. Of the 308 adult index cases, 208 were married; 130 of them had children (a total of 352) of whom 11 had congenital heart defects. Thus, an average of one child affected with a congenital heart defect was born to every 12 patients in this series who had children.

The data were analyzed to determine whether or not the percentage of affected children of parents with congenital heart defects approximates the prediction of the multifactorial inheritance hypothesis for the etiology of congenital heart diseases.[1] The incidence in first-degree relatives of an individual with a malformation transmitted by multifactorial inheritance approaches the square root of the population frequency of that lesion. For ASD the 2.6% of offspring affected is precisely the multifactorial prediction, and for VSD the 3.7% of children with cardiac malformations closely approximates the 4.2% prediction. These figures for ASD and VSD are based on patients personally examined (or autopsy

122

Table 1.—Adults With ASD* or VSD† (Total No., 308)

	No. With ASD		No. With VSD		
	Female	Male	Female	Male	Total No.
Total No. of patients	108	59	67	74	308
Married patients	68	44	44	52	208
Patients with children	42	31	25	32	130
No. of children	121	69	71	91	352
Male children	59	35	36	44	174
Female children	62	34	35	47	178
No. of children with congenital heart disease	2	3	4	2	11

*ASD indicates atrial-septal defect.
†VSD indicates ventricular-septal defect.

Table 2.—Adults, Married, Ages 20-29 Years

	Ages (%)	
	20-24	25-29
Women		
National (1967)	67.6	86.3
This study	31	59
Men		
National (1967)		81.4
This study		64

records) and represent the minimum recurrence risk in this series. Because of the difficulty in detecting a small atrial-septal defect in young children, it is possible that some patients, examined by their physicians and considered not to have an ASD, may have the lesion.

All affected offspring of parents with ASD had ASD alone or in combination with other defects such as pulmonic stenosis or pulmonary valve atresia. The affected children of parents with VSD all had VSD as an isolated lesion or in association with other cardiovascular anomalies. The associated malformations were patent ductus arteriosus and coarctation of the aorta in one patient and pulmonic stenosis in another child.

An effort was made to determine the fertility of patients with congenital heart malformations in order to gain some estimate as to the possibility that we are increasing the incidence of these lesions by therapeutic intervention, but our sample proved too small to compare directly with national fertility rates. However, if one cannot accurately determine fertility rates in so small a sample, certain data may serve as a potential indicator of fertility. Table 2 suggests that patients with congenital heart lesions have a marriage pattern which differs from that of the general population. Patients with heart defects appear to marry later, and the percentage of those marrying by age 30 (and perhaps by any age) is apparently lower than that of the American population in 1967.[2] This trend could be responsible for a lower fertility rate.

Comment

Patients with ASD have a frequency of this lesion in their children of 2.6%, which is 37 times higher than the estimated population prevalence of 0.07%.[3] This 2.6% frequency falls far short of a Mendelian expectation but is precisely the expectation of multifactorial inheritance. It is therefore proposed that 2.6% may be used in genetic counseling as an empirical risk figure for the *first* occurrence of ASD in the offspring of a parent with ASD. This applies to the first occurrence only, because in multifactorial inheritance the occurrence risk increases precipitously with the number of affected first-degree relatives.

Ventricular-septal defect occurs in 3.7% of the offspring of parents with VSD, which closely approximates the 4.2% multifactorial inheritance expectation, and is 21 times the 0.175% estimated general prevalence of VSD.[1] For the purposes of genetic counseling, the empirical risk figure of 3.7% is proposed for the first occurrence of VSD in the child of a parent with VSD.

It is of interest that there is a high degree of concordance in the affected offspring of parents with ASD and VSD, supporting the contention that these lesions should be evaluated as separate diseases and not simply lumped together as "congenital heart disease."[4]

We have now had the first marriage on our service between patients, each with VSD, and we are receiving further inquiries for counseling of patients considering marriage who have become acquainted while undergoing diagnostic examination, surgery, and follow-up examinations. The possibility of a high incidence of affected offspring from such marriages is portended by the recognized increased risk in families in which more than one first-degree relative is affected (which presumably reflects the segregation of an increased number of genes predisposing to the defect). This increased risk has been demonstrated in another congenital malformation presumably conforming to multifactorial inheritance—cleft lip and palate.[5] Preliminary data sup-

124

porting an increased risk with increasing number of affected first-degree relatives have been obtained in ASD.[3]

Although the rate of occurrence of heart lesions in the offspring of patients with VSD and ASD is 21 to 37 times greater than the population frequency, the larger social question of whether recent therapeutic advances will gradually increase the prevalence of congenital heart lesions cannot be answered on the basis of this small sample. It is possible that diminished fertility may still be offsetting some of the potential for reproducing congenital heart lesions in subsequent generations. At present, it appears that patients who have had operative repair of congenital heart lesions, and hence should not have significant physical incapacity, are not marrying as early or as frequently as the general population, and thus may be voluntarily diminishing their fertility rate and decreasing the chance of transmitting the tendency toward congenital heart disease. However, an increasingly large number of patients with congenital heart defects who would not have survived into reproductive age are now reproducing.

The implications for the individual parent with a cardiac anomaly regarding the emotional and financial stress imposed by having a child with a congenital heart lesion are presented, and the very personal decision of parenthood may be based on the empirical risks thus far demonstrated. The broader social implications must yet be determined.

This investigation was supported by grants from the National Foundation, the Texas Heart Institute, and by Public Health Service grant HE-5756 from the National Institutes of Health.

References

1. Nora, J.J.: Multifactorial Inheritance Hypothesis for the Etiology of Congenital Heart Diseases: The Genetic-Environmental Interaction, Circulation 38:604-617 (Sept) 1968.

2. Statistical Abstract of the United States: 1967, ed 88, Washington, 1967, p 33.

3. Nora, J.J.; McNamara, D.G.; and Fraser, F.C.: Hereditary Factors in Atrial Septal Defect, Circulation 35:448-456 (March) 1967.

4. Nora, J.J., and Meyer, T.C.: Familial Nature of Congenital Heart Diseases, Pediatrics 37:329-334 (Feb) 1966.

5. Curtis, E.; Fraser, F.C.; and Warburton, D.: Congenital Cleft Lip and Palate: Risk Figures for Counseling, Amer J Dis Child 102:853-857 (Dec) 1961.

COMMON MALFORMATIONS OF THE HEART

By MAURICE CAMPBELL

It is well recognized in human genetics that the manifestation of clinical disease depends on the interplay between genetic and environmental factors. A good example of this is hereditary spherocytosis. In a family of 67 persons the condition was present in 13 out of 34 examined in three generations (Campbell 1921) and in a mother and grandmother of the earlier generation. The condition seemed to be inherited as a dominant autosomal Mendelian character, though this was at first uncertain because at least two subjects who had transmitted the condition appeared normal and had never been recognized as jaundiced. When, however, their blood was examined their red cells were found to be abnormal—being haemolysed by $0 \cdot 6$ per cent. saline instead of the normal $0 \cdot 45$ per cent. It was the abnormality of the red cells that was inherited as a strictly dominant character, but whether there was enough haemolysis to produce overt jaundice depended on environmental factors. Two recent reviews of this subject (Dacie 1954, Young 1955) accept the method of inheritance as dominant but with wide variation in its expression, only about a quarter instead of a half of the sibs being affected.

The pattern of a genetic background with an added environmental factor seems to be the most common cause of malformations of the heart. Between 1955 and 1964 we have been able to report findings in the families of 1,227 patients with the commoner malformations of the heart. These findings have been published (Campbell 1965). The main conclusions reached can be summarized.

(1) Children with a malformation of the heart are more likely to have a second malformation of the heart than would be expected by chance. They are also more likely to have a non-cardiac malformation.

(2) More of the sibs of the propositi, 2 per cent. instead of $0 \cdot 6$ per cent., have a malformation of the heart. This is important for genetic counselling since it is not very likely that another child will have a malformation of the heart though more likely than in the general population.

(3) The parents of the propositi are not, in general, more likely to have a cardiac malformation, perhaps because those

who have are less likely to have children. An exception is in some families with atrial septal defect (ASD) where dominant Mendelian inheritance seems to be the rule.

(4) Probably the children of those with malformations of the heart are more likely to have such malformations, but more evidence is needed to be sure of this. Neill and Swanson (1961) found an incidence of 1·8 per cent. of children with a heart malformation in 508 pregnancies where one parent had such a malformation, substantially the same as the incidence in sibs of the propositi.

TABLE I

CONSANGUINITY OF PARENTS OF PROPOSITI WITH MALFORMATIONS OF THE HEART

	Percentage of parents who were first cousins (Campbell 1965)	Index of consanguinity		
		Campbell (1965)	Lamy et al. (1957)	Mean
P.D.A. ..	1·6	1·6	2·3	1·9
A.S.D. ..	1·9	2·4	3·8	3·1
V.S.D. ..	1·2	1·4	0·9	1·2
Coarct. ..	0	0	0·6	0·3
P.V.S. ..	0·9	0·9	4·5	2·7
Fallot's ..	0·8	1·0	0·1	0·6
Mean ..	1·1	1·2	2·0	1·6
Normal ..	0·4–0·5	—	0·7	0·6
Situs inversus ..	5·3*	5·6	14·3	—

* These are taken from 379 families and include reported as well as personal cases (Campbell 1963).

(5) The malformation found in the sibs is 15 times as likely to be concordant (the same or similar) as would be expected by chance. This is also true for parents with ASD, and may be for the children of propositi, but the evidence for this is still inadequate.

(6) The incidence of first-cousin marriages among the parents of our propositi is greater than expected in the general population. The figures for the different malformations are shown in Table I, and the index makes an allowance for second-cousin marriages also (Lamy's index is calculated rather differently from mine). Possibly coarctation of the aorta does not show this increased consanguinity, but the numbers are not large enough to prove this.

For most malformations of the heart the rate is three times as high as among the general population, which is enough to point to the importance of a recessive Mendelian factor. For *situs inversus* it is more than ten times as high.

127

(7) Maternal age does not appear of much importance though rather more children with malformations of the heart were born to mothers aged 35 or over. After excluding all children with mongolism (because of the known effect of maternal age) significantly more children with Fallot's tetralogy were born to mothers aged 40 and over. Significantly more sixth and later children with ventricular septal defect (VSD) were born to mothers aged 35–39 and the excess born to mothers 35 and over only just failed to reach the level of statistical significance. In other groups it was not certain that the excess was significant.

(8) Penrose (1955) pointed out that the difference between the *means of the paternal and maternal ages* is in some ways a more useful measurement, since an undue increase of the paternal age suggests the possibility of a "failure to copy genes correctly because of the larger number of cell divisions in the male germline".

The mean paternal age exceeded the mean maternal age by more than expected in each group. In coarctation the excess was only 6 per cent., probably not significant, but in all the others it was 17 per cent. or more. This is another pointer to a genetic factor, though the average excess of 3·3 years is much less than that found in achondroplasia, 5·6 years (Penrose 1957) and 7·2 years (Stevenson 1957).

(9) Children with malformations of the heart tend to be lighter at birth than their normal sibs. But the difference is significant only for girls with coarctation and for girls and boys with ventricular septal defect.

(10) An unusual seasonal incidence of conception may indicate the influence of an environmental factor. McKeown and Record (1951) and Edwards (1958) found that the births of those with anencephaly were more frequent in the two winter quarters. Rutstein, Nickerson and Heald (1952), in America, found more births of subjects with patent ductus arteriosus (PDA) from October to January.

Record and McKeown (1953), in Birmingham, found a seasonal incidence for girls with PDA but not for boys. My figures agree with theirs. Combining them, more affected girls were born from May to November with a peak in August, but the boys were more equally distributed. Our figures for some other cardiac malformations (Campbell 1965) show some differences but they are variable and need the support of larger numbers before any valid conclusions can be reached.

(11) The proportion of male subjects with the various common malformations of the heart at birth ranges from 40 per cent. with

TABLE II
CHROMOSOMAL ABNORMALITIES

TRISOMY
(1) Chromos. 21. Mongolism with septal defects and A–V canal defects.
(2) Chr. (17) or 18.   V.S.D. (20 of 22), flexed fingers, and small mandibles.
(3) Chr. 13–15.   V.S.D. (9 of 15), deafness, hare-lip, and polydactyly.
In both (2) and (3) mentally-retarded and deformed ears.
SEX CHROMOSOME
Turner's syndrome, often with coarctation of aorta.

PDA to 73 per cent. with transposition of the great trunks. This must be connected with the aetiology of these conditions in some way, but we do not know how. There is also a selective mortality, so that the sex incidence changes from birth to adult life.

Many of these findings are similar to the conclusions of Neel (1960) about several non-cardiac malformations.

Some conclusions can be drawn about the causation from these and other observations and from experiments on animals.

Chromosomal abnormalities. No malformations of the heart are known to be caused in this way solely, but they are frequently present in conditions that are so caused. These are listed in Table II. The malformations, especially septal defects, found with mongolism due to trisomy of chromosome 21, and those, especially coarctation, found with Turner's syndrome (Campbell and Polani 1961a) due to an XO sex chromosome are both common; but the others are rare conditions.

Dominant Mendelian inheritance. This seems to be the main cause only in many groups of familial cardiomyopathy and the aortic defects associated with Marfan's syndrome (Table III). A most striking family with the former condition was described by Paré, Fraser, Pirozynski, Shanks and Stubington (1961), going back to the seventeenth century.

A few cases with atrial septal defect or with aortic stenosis have a familial incidence with dominant inheritance (Campbell and Polani 1961b). A family tree with ASD is shown in Figure 1. There are two cases where the ASD may have been passed through

TABLE III
DOMINANT MENDELIAN INHERITANCE

1. Familial cardiomyopathy.
   Special form with naevi, dwarfism and E.E.C. changes (Polani, Moynihan).
2. Arachnodactyly (Marfan's syndrome).
   Defects of aortic valve and aorta (rupture).
3. *Some cases* of A.S.D. and perhaps aortic stenosis.
4. *Some cases* of cardiac arrhythmias.

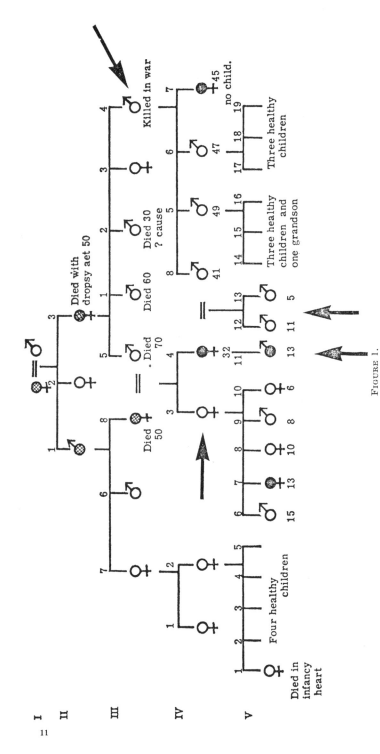

FIGURE 1.

A family tree showing 4 proved and 4 probable cases of atrial septal defect. The inheritance was probably dominant, but the upper arrows indicate two patients who transmitted the condition though they themselves were not proved to have an A.S.D. For the lower arrows indicating the children of IV 4 who herself had A.S.D., see text.

a parent who was not affected, but otherwise the inheritance was dominant with rather low penetrance. It is interesting that the illegitimate child of IV 4 inherited the condition from her, but when she married her first cousin she bore him two normal children.

Recessive Mendelian inheritance. This is much more important as the main cause of *situs inversus* in man (Cockayne 1938, Torgersen 1950, Campbell 1963) and as a partial cause of most malformations of the heart (Table IV). The high proportion of cousin

TABLE IV
RECESSIVE MENDELIAN INHERITANCE

1. *Situs inversus* in Man.
2. S.I. (a) in 57 of 227 offspring from inbreeding in a strain of *mice* (Tihen *et. al.* 1948)
   (b) in 37% of an inbred strain of *platyfish* (Baker-Cohen 1961)
3. V.S.D. (288 cases) in *fowls*—97% in 3 inbred lines in which 84, 50 and 30% affected (Siller 1958)

Of much more general importance as a *partial cause* in most malformations of the heart.

marriages, 10 times normal for *situs inversus* and nearly three times normal for all other malformations, is one part of the evidence. The excess of mean paternal age is another.

The malformation of the heart in 2 per cent. of the sibs of propositi could be due to environmental causes. But the high degree of concordance between the malformations in the propositus and the sib (60 per cent. the same and another 20 per cent. partially so) can be more readily understood if the cause is genetic.

Recessive inheritance is not, however, the whole cause since it is unusual for both of a pair of monozygotic twins to be affected (Uchida and Rowe 1957, Campbell 1961). They are, however, both affected more often than other pairs of twins (Fuhrmann 1958).

There is further support for this view from animal breeding experiments. Tihen, Charles and Sippel (1948) found by inbreeding a particular strain of laboratory mice that 57 of 227 had *situs inversus*. Baker-Cohen (1961) found it in 37 per cent. of an inbred strain of the platyfish though it was rare or absent in most strains of this or related sword-tails. Further, Siller (1958) found 288 examples of ventricular septal defect in fowl, and 97 per cent. of these were confined to three inbred lines in which 84, 50 and 30 per cent. were affected. All these workers thought their findings pointed to recessive inheritance, sometimes with incomplete expression.

131

Environmental causes. Maternal rubella in the first trimester of pregnancy is practically alone in being established as a cause of malformations of the heart, especially PDA. But it cannot account for much more than 2 per cent. of the total.

Many other causes are thought to have caused a few cases. Of other viral infections, a few cases caused by measles, chicken-pox, whooping cough, herpes zoster, infectious hepatitis, mumps, poliomyelitis, and other viruses have been seen. But considering the interest that has been taken in the subject, it seems most unlikely that any of them cause malformations on a scale comparable with rubella. Threatened abortions can be suspected as a cause but are very difficult to assess without a prospective study carefully planned and on a large scale.

Much of the experimental work on animals has shown that many malformations, including sometimes but not often those of the heart, can be produced by the most varied causes by deficiency of oxygen or of riboflavin, by injections of cortisone or insulin, and by boric acid and many other substances. Hog-cholera vaccines given to sows in early pregnancy have produced abortions and several malformations (but not of the heart), and similar results have been seen with blue-tongue virus in sheep (Rhodes 1960).

Mother rats kept on diets deficient in vitamin A gave birth to offspring with malformations of the aortic arches, bulbus, and ventricular septum (Wilson and Warkany 1949, Wilson, Roth and Warkany 1953). The poor diet of many mothers a generation ago might have led to such malformations but the vast improvement that has taken place in this direction without any reduction in the incidence of malformations is evidence against this being a significant cause in man.

The interplay of genetic and environmental factors in the experimental production of malformations by teratogens has been emphasized increasingly. Many workers have found that different strains reacted very differently to the same teratogenic agent; that a particular malformation might be produced only in one or a few strains; and that many malformations were apt to occur in a particular strain without any teratogen, though then only on much smaller numbers. Campbell (1965) quoted many examples from Landauer (1945, 1952, 1953), Kalter (1954), Kalter and Warkany (1957), and others, so they need not be repeated here.

SUMMARY

Few malformations of the heart in man can be attributed to single genes or to other known genetic or environmental factors

132

acting alone. *Situs inversus* has been quoted as an example where recessive Mendelian inheritance is of special importance, and in a few families with cardiomyopathy or atrial septal defect dominant inheritance has been important.

Maternal rubella in the first trimester of pregnancy is the best established environmental cause. It is not, however, responsible for much more than 2 per cent. of all malformations of the heart.

Recessive Mendelian inheritance is of more general importance in most malformations of the heart, but not as the sole cause.

Foxon (1959) wrote: "A zygote will develop into a normal animal if its genetic constitution is normal, and if the environment in which development takes place is normal." A few examples where a malformation of the heart is produced by one of these causes alone have been given. But more generally some recessive genetic factor is of considerable importance but is effective only under certain environmental conditions. Lamy, de Grouchy and Schweisguth (1957) in France and Fuhrmann (1961, 1962) in Germany are in general agreement with these views.

Probably the development of the heart is governed by a multifactorial system with a balance of many interacting genes. Any change in this balance, e.g. an increase of homozygosity, may cause a breakdown so that exogenous factors, normally rendered harmless by the self-regulation, can lead to malformations.

REFERENCES

Baker-Cohen, K. F. (1961) *Amer. J. Anat.*, **109**, 37.
Campbell, M. (1921) *Guy's Hospital Rep.*, **71**, 274.
Campbell, M. (1961) *Acta Genet. med. (Roma)*, **10**, 443.
Campbell, M. (1963) *Brit. Heart J.*, **25**, 803.
Campbell, M. (1965) *Brit. med. J.*, **ii**, 895.
Campbell, M. and Polani, P. E. (1961a) *Lancet*, **i**, 463.
Campbell, M. and Polani, P. E. (1961b) *Brit. Heart J.*, **23**, 477.
Cockayne, E. A. (1938) *Quart. J. Med.*, **7**, 479.
Dacie, J. V. (1954) *The Haemolytic Anaemias: Congenital and Acquired.* J. & A. Churchill, London.
Edwards, J. H. (1958) *Brit. J. prev. soc. Med.*, **12**, 115.
Foxon, G. E. H. (1959) *Brit. Heart J.*, **21**, 51.
Fuhrmann, W. (1958) *Z. menshl. Vererb, u. Konstit.—Lehre*, **34**, 563.
Fuhrmann, W. (1961) *Acta genet. (Basel)*, **11**, 289.
Fuhrmann, W. (1962) *Ergebn. inn. Med. Kinderheilk*, **18**, 47.
Kalter, H. (1954) *Genetics*, **39**, 185 and 975.
Kalter, H. and Warkany, J. (1957) *J. exp. Zool.*, **136**, 531.
Lamy, M., de Grouchy, J. and Schweisguth, O. (1957) *Amer. J. hum. Genet.*, **9**, 17.
Landauer, W (1945) *J. exp. Zool.*, **98**, 1.
Landauer, W. (1952) *J. exp. Zool.*, **120**, 469.
Landauer, W. (1953) *Genetics*, **38**, 216.
McKeown, T. and Record, R. G. (1951) *Lancet*, **i**, 192.
Neel, J. V. (1960) In *First International Conference on Congenital Malformations*, p. 63. Pitman, London, 1962.
Neill, Catherine and Swanson, S. (1961) *Circulation*, **24**, 1003.
Paré, J. A. P., Fraser, R. G., Pirozynski, W. J., Shanks, J. A. and Stubington, D. (1961) *Amer. J. Med.*, **31**, 37.
Penrose, L. S. (1955) *Lancet*, **ii**, 312.
Penrose, L. S. (1957) *Amer J. hum. Genet.*, **9**, 167.

Record, R. G. and McKeown, T. (1953) *Brit. Heart J.*, **15**, 376.
Rhodes, A. J. (1960) In *First International Conference on Congenital Malformations*, p. 106. Pitman, London, 1962.
Rutstein, D. D., Nickerson, R. J. and Heald, F. P. (1952) *Amer. J. Dis. Child.*, **84**, 199.
Siller, W. G. (1958) *J. Path. Bact.*, **76**, 431.
Stevenson, A. C. (1957) *Amer. J. hum. Genet.*, **9**, 81.
Tihen, J. A., Charles, D. R. and Sippel, T. O. (1948) *J. Hered.*, **39**, 29.
Torgersen, J. (1950) *Amer. J. hum. Genet.*, **2**, 361.
Uchida, Irene A. and Rowe, R. D. (1957) *Amer. J. hum. Genet.*, **9**, 133.
Wilson, J. G. and Warkany, J. (1949) *Amer. J. Anat.*, **85**, 113.
Wilson, J. G., Roth, C. B. and Warkany, J. (1953) *Amer. J. Anat.*, **92**, 189.
Young, L. E. (1955) *Amer. J. Med.*, **18**, 486.

MICROTIC, LOP, CUP AND PROTRUDING EARS:

FOUR DIRECTLY INHERITABLE DEFORMITIES?

BLAIR O. ROGERS, M.D.

"Small pitchers have wyde eares"
   (*John Heywoode,*[1] *1598*)

"The Ears . . . have been framed by the Providence of Nature into two twining passages like a Snails shell . . . "
   (*Ambroise Paré,*[2] *1678*)

"In certain degenerates, and also in some apparently normal individuals, the contour of the auricles is abnormal. In an accentuated form we find the so called "lop ears" and in the less marked conditions the appearance of the Darwinian tubercle"
   (*John Staige Davis,*[3] *1919*)

Wyde ears! Snail shell ears! Degenerate ears! Lost ears![4] Whorléd ears![5] With the exception of the connotation of "degeneracy," innocently perpetuated by the great John Staige Davis[3] almost 50 years ago, the other adjectives cited above are relatively mild and benign. Let us, for example, peruse an alphabetical list of some of the more descriptive, often cruel and frequently inaccurate adjectives employed by both laymen and physicians over the past century with equal abandon.

"Bat" ears, "big" ears, "cat" . . ., cercopithicus . . ., clown, cup, devil's, dog, donkey, droopy, Dumbo, elephant, elf, flap, flop, folded, jug, lap-dog, lop, Macacus, Machiavellian, Mephistophelean, monkey, Mozart, obtrusive, pitcher, pixie, pointed, projecting, prominent, protuberant, protruding, rabbit, radar, "red sails in the sunset," ridge, sail, Satan, satyr, shell, spaniel, Stahl's, "taxi with wide open doors," teacup, triangular, and Wildermuth's ears.

135

Despite this long and diverse list of adjectives, however, these more than 40 descriptive terms offer little help to the clinician who wishes to more accurately describe the major external ear deformities to his colleagues. For the purposes of reducing this descriptive terminology to a minimum, therefore, and because they are terms and/or deformities which appear in the literature with the greatest frequency, it will be proposed here that there are only 4 chief external ear deformities which encompass most, if not all of the above list of more than 40 terms—namely microtia, lop ears, cup ears, and protruding ears. Their major physical characteristics may be described as follows.

TYPES OF DEFORMITIES

1. Microtia: a distinctly malformed and underdeveloped auricle, always smaller in size (Fig. 14*I*) than the normal unaffected external ear, with (Fig. 14*I*) or without (Fig. 14*A*) some of the characteristic features of the normal auricle. In the majority of cases, only rudimentary or imperfectly developed remnants exist; these may take the form of a malformed lobule, with the rest of the pinna being totally or almost completely absent (Fig. 14*A*) and complete atresia of the canal, or a malformed pinna (any portion, half, third, or quarter of) which survives with or without a malformed lobule (Fig. 14*G*, *H*), or a series of vestigial remnants which are similar to the "hillocks" (Fig. 14*B*, *C*, *D*, *E*, *F*) seen in the 6th week of embryonic development of the external ear.

2. Lop Ear: a malformed auricle in which the characteristic major deformity consists of an acute downward folding and/or deficiency of the helix and scapha (Figs. 15*E*, 20*I*), usually at the level of the tuberculum auriculae (Darwin's tubercle) in association with a malformation or inadequate development or deficiency of the antihelix (more

136

commonly at the superior crus). In some cases the downward folding or flattening of the superior pole of the pinna may lie at a level slightly above the tuberculum auriculae (Fig. 15F) and thus give the physical illusion of a more nearly normal auricle. (The ears of South African Bushmen are characteristicly square or flattened on top, as well as being small and often lobeless.[6]) In other cases, the lopping (which actually implies "limpness") may occur below the tuberculum auriculae (Figs. 15B, 20H) to create a microtia–like deformity in which the lopped superior portion of the ear hangs so limply, or droops to such a degree, that it covers or hides the anterior, concave surface of the concha in the manner of a hood or a drawn window-shade.

Because some lop ears may appear smaller than normal, some authors have categorized these deformities as variants of microtia (Fig. 20E, F).

Similarly, some lop ears have been termed cup ears by those authors who pay less attention to the faulty development of the downward, folded, or compressed, or flattened superior helix-scaphal-antihelix region, and pay more attention to any exaggerated cupping, or over-development, of the concha. Obviously there are gradations between microtia and "lopping," just as there are gradations between lopping and cupping, in all of these many and varied expressions of the embryologic and fetal maldevelopment of the auricle.

3. *Cup Ear:* an essentially malformed protruding ear which has characteristics of both lop ears and protruding ears. The cup ear protrudes because of the exaggerated over-development of its deep, "cup-shaped", concave concha. The deficient or faulty development of the superior half (or third or quarter) of its helix margin and antihelical crura is in keeping with some of the characteristics of a lop

ear (Figs. 2C, 16A, B, C, D, and 21B, C, D, E, F, G, H). As a result of this deficiency in most cup ears, and the occasional cupping forward of the lobule, the height of the ear from the top of the superior pole to the bottom of the lobule seems to be, or is, reduced. The usually encountered cup ear thus seems to be slightly smaller than normal (Figs 16A, B, C, D) in its vertical height as contrasted with the protruding ear, which almost always seems to be normal, or even slightly larger than normal, in size. In addition, the often wider, unfurled helix margin combined with a frequently unformed, or poorly developed, body of the antihelix exaggerates the cupping deformity. In some cases, the helix margin, or fold, cups forward and over the scapha as a hood (Figs. 16A, 21E, G).

Thus, in following the reasoning briefly described in a previous section (see lop ear), the cup ear would seem to represent a stage of development or maldevelopment which lies between the lop ear and the protruding ear.

It is interesting that when one "cups one's ear" to better hear a speaker or an indistinctly heard sound, one physically reproduces in his normal ear and its lobule the cup ear deformity. Perhaps this is another explanation of how this term entered the medical literature.

4. Protruding Ear: a protruding ear approximates the normal ear in its shape and size, with the exception of several major characteristics that may represent arrested development. The usual protruding ear has a normal vertical height, as contrasted to the smaller lop and cup ears, but one chief anatomical maldevelopment, or a combination of several malformations, contribute to its protrusion. These may include:

(a). An unfurled and/or poorly formed body of the antihelix (Fig. 22C, D) or antihelical crura (Fig. 2A) or both (Fig. 22B).

138

(b). Excessive conchal cartilage (Figs. 16*E*, 21*H*, *I*).

(c). Increased angle of protrusion of the lobule and/or excess lobule size (Figs. 21*I*, 22*E*).

(d). Inadequate folding of the helix margin or "shell" ear (Figs. 21*F*, 22*G*). The thin, unrolled margin of a "shell" ear resembles the thin edge of a clam shell, which probably explains this descriptive term.

It is not the purpose of this paper to describe other deformities of the external ear region such as pre-auricular fistulae, pits, and/or appendages, or meatal atresia, but instead to correct some of the misinterpreted information concerning the four external ear deformities described above. Some long-standing facts about the external ear, for example, are not "*facts*" at all, but mere bits and smidgens of unscientific hearsay.

John Staige Davis,[3] therefore, was merely repeating the long held, but erroneous, pseudo-anthropologic belief that criminals, "degenerates," and the criminally insane have abnormalities of the external ear as abnormal as their social behavior. This belief was certainly not lessened by Ernest Hooton of Harvard, who in his book *Crime and the Man*,[7] stated that the ears of criminals more often demonstrated unrolled helical margins, more frequent, well-developed Darwin's tubercles, and shorter, broader, more "primitive" proportions. This type of thinking, supported by poorly controlled anthropologic data and measurements, was probably an outgrowth of the Bertillon system. For many years in several European countries this system was taught to police officers, suggesting that they memorize the morphologic variations of the external ear as clues to criminal identification as well as to criminal tendencies. Although an ear photograph could be used as a form of finger-printing the criminal, one readily understands how one may completely upset this form of identification merely by performing a **corrective otoplasty.**

External ear characteristics have been helpful in some problems of paternity diagnosis[8] but anatomical features of the auricle have a very complex genetic basis, which undoubtedly involves many genes. Among anatomical characteristics studied in some cases of paternity diagnosis are ear mass, outline, position, curl and course of the helix, breadth and convexity of the antihelix, convexity of the tragus and antitragus, form of the incisura intertragica, and the attachment and prominence of the ear lobule.[8]

A genetic basis for the shape of the external ear is obvious, but the inheritance of specific differences in both normal and abnormal characteristics of the auricle has been described only during the past half–century. Now it can be stated that large ears are "dominant" over small ears,[9] that Darwin's tubercle is inherited as a dominant trait,[10] and that free ear lobes seem to be dominant over attached ear lobes.[10] One might ask, therefore, what are the other facts pertinent to the inheritance of ear deformities which have been verified within recent decades?

HEREDITARY FACTORS

In 1921, Siemens[11] reported the probable inheritance of *pre-auricular appendages* in members of the same family; he also reviewed other cases which had appeared in the literature prior to his report, demonstrating an inherited factor in this disorder.

Also in the year 1921, Kindred[12] uncovered a family with a history of *auricular fistulae* or *pits* in 4 generations, an example of irregular dominance. This was substantiated by Quelprud,[13] who in 1940 investigated the irregular expression of this dominance in a family of 150 persons.

Ruttin,[14] in 1927, demonstrated the separate appearance of *auricular fistulae* and *auricular appendages* in different members of the same family.

In 1937, Powell and Whitney[15] demonstrated, in 2 families studied for 3 successive generations, that *free ear lobes* are inherited as dominant characters and that *adherent ear lobes* are recessives.

In 1937, Potter[16] reported a family of 92 persons in whom *cup ears*, invariably bilateral and more severe in their abnormal shape than protruding ears, were inherited by 23 members of the family over a span of 5 generations, thus demonstrating a regular dominance in the action of the offending gene in this disorder. Normal siblings in this family, however, who married normal persons did not transmit this cup ear defect to their offspring.

In an extensive review in 1939, Brander[17] stated that geneologic studies previously reported in the literature, together with his own findings, demonstrated beyond doubt that *auricular appendages* ". . . are at any rate to some extent hereditarily conditioned. Many circumstances seem to speak in favor of the fact that it may be here the question of a dominant pre-disposition with variegated penetration." [17]

In 1949, Hanhart[18] reported a simple, uncomplicated, mild form of *microtia* which was inherited, according to regular dominance of the genetic effect, with a 100 per cent "penetrance" in 7 generations and in 5 generations of 2 different families, respectively, without any lapse or skip in the inheritance of the defect. These 2 families thus represented a total of 64 carriers of this type of mild microtia. Hanhart also reported a more severe form of inheritable *microtia* in which only a very rudimentary development of the concha was evident, combined with atresia of the canal and cleft or abnormally high palates. This syndrome appeared much less frequently than the milder form of microtia and, in the affected families studied, the involvement of only 4 members of a family of 40 demonstrated that the genetic effect was one of irregular dominance with very feeble penetrance.

In a recent paper, Wildervanck[19] (in 1962) described a family in which *protruding ears, lop ears, pre-auricular tabs, pre-auricular marginal pits, microtia,* and/or conductive deafness occurred in several members of a family in whom these deformities were present in 3 generations. Thus, the dominant role of heredity in the etiology of these ear anomalies in this family is evident, although a study of each generation reveals that the expression of these various types of inherited ear deformities is very inconstant.

In 1964, Rogers[20] described 2 members of a Puerto Rican family (see Fig. 1) showing a hereditary pre-disposition for ear deformities. In one, a 12-year-old boy, a partial *microtia* of the right ear and a relative protruding conchal deformity of the left ear could be observed. In his 10-year-old brother, bilateral *protruding* ears were demonstrable. The importance of heredity in cases of protruding ears, cases uncomplicated by any major or minor degree of microtia in any other members of the family, can be seen in Figure 2, which reveals the protruding ears of a 39-year-old father, 2 of whose 3 children have severely protruding ears, and 1 of whom has ears which are more properly termed as lopped "cup" ears.

The obvious hereditary basis of many of these ear deformities, as outlined in the above brief review of the literature, demonstrates that in any given family with these inheritance patterns, there is a variable expression of these anomalies. This suggests that there might very well be critical phases in embryologic development which determine whether one or another or a combination of these anomalies will eventually appear at birth as "post-facto" clinical evidence of arrested stages of embryologic, or fetal, development of the ear. We must next ask ourselves, "What morphologic relationship, if any, exists be-

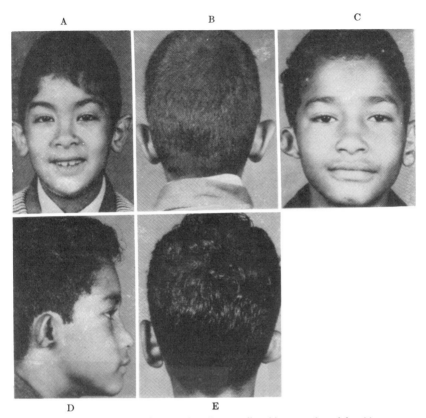

Fig. 1. Members of a family showing a hereditary predisposition toward ear deformities, seen at our clinic. (*A, B*) 10-year-old boy with bilateral protuberant ears. (*C–E*) 12-year-old brother demonstrating relative protruding conchal deformity of left ear and partial microtia of right ear. (From Rogers, B. O., in *Reconstructive Plastic Surgery*, edited by J. M. Converse. Vol. III, p. 1213. W. B. Saunders Co., Philadelphia. 1964.)

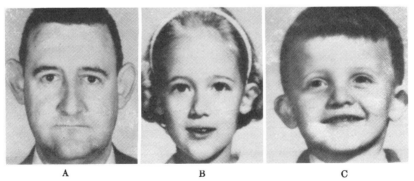

Fig. 2. (*A*) Father, 39-year-old, with markedly protruding ears; (*B*) daughter, 8-year-old, with similar protruding ears, and (*C*) son, 5-year-old, with slightly lopped "cup" ears.

143

tween microtia, lop ears, cup ears, protruding ears, and the so-called "normal" embryologic-fetal development of the external ear?"

VARIABLE GENETIC PENETRANCE

A probable relationship between microtia, lop ears, cup ears, and protruding ear deformities became increasingly evident to me earlier last year. At that time I had been rapidly thumbing through the photographs of several hundred cases of ear deformities which have been operated upon in the Department of Plastic Surgery of the Manhattan Eye, Ear and Throat Hospital, to make a more accurate diagnosis of these cases for an IBM card system. (It was at this same hospital, 87 years ago, in 1881, that Dr. Edward T. Ely[30] of New York performed what was probably the first operation for the correction of protruding ears in the New World.)

It soon became apparent to me that microtia, lop ears, cup ears, and protruding ear deformities often shared some physical characteristics more frequently than they differed from each other, or appeared, as isolated distinct entities. As an example of this, Figures 15–17 and 20–22 demonstrate some of the marked variations in overall contour of lop ears, cup ears, and protruding ears, variations which differ as much from the standard normal ear as one expects to find in the more obvious cases of true microtia with its variations (Figs. 14, 18, 19, 20).

In trying to formulate a hypothesis which would demonstrate the overlapping relationship of these deformities, it was necessary to find a hereditary deformity of the first and second branchial arches in which any one of these ear deformities could be present or absent, depending upon what geneticists call the "variable" expression, or the degrees of "penetrance," of the offending gene or genes involved in their etiology. This is to say, that

144

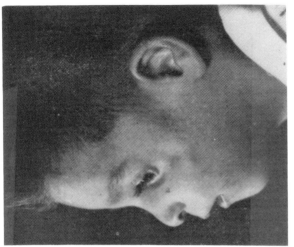

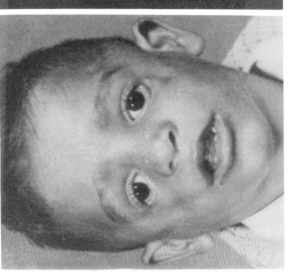

FIG. 3. Photographs of a 4-year-old boy, demonstrating the "incomplete" form of mandibulo-facial dysostosis with normal. slightly protruding ears—otherwise obvious as a typical case of "Treacher Collins syndrome," as it is understood by British and American authorities. These photographs demonstrate anti-mongoloid obliquity or slant of the palpebral fissures, unilateral notching of the left lower eyelid, deficiency or absence of the eyelashes of the medial two-thirds of the lower eyelids, and malar hypoplasia. (From Rogers, B. O.: Berry-Treacher Collins syndrome: a review of 200 cases. Brit. J. Plast. Surg., *17:* 109, 1964.)

any individual afflicted with this hereditary deformity or syndrome should have at least one of 4 or 5 different types of ears as a possible physical characteristic, namely—"normal," "protruding," "cup," "lop," or "microtic" ears. The disorder which meets these hypothetical requirements does exist and is known as the Berry-Treacher-Collins syndrome, or mandibulofacial dysostosis (Figs. 18F, 19C, D). This syndrome is transmitted in many cases by an irregularly dominant gene, whose power of expression is variable and sometimes weak in its penetrance, thus resulting in "incomplete" or "abortive" types of the syndrome in which the ears may be normal (or almost normal) as far as the external ear is concerned, even though deafness may often be present (see Fig. 3). The cases originally described by Treacher-Collins belong to the *incomplete* form of mandibulofacial dysostosis.

When the gene has an apparently "strong" degree of penetrance, however, a more *complete* and severe form of the syndrome may occur in which a severe malformation of the external ears, such as microtia, is often seen, as well as deformities of the middle and inner ears (see Figs. 18F, 19C, D). Having established the variable genetic expressiveness of ear deformities in more than 200 cases of the Berry-Treacher-Collins syndrome,[21] it next becomes necessary to understand their onset and development by reviewing the events that occur in early embryologic and fetal development of the external ear.

EMBRYOLOGIC-FETAL DEVELOPMENT OF THE EXTERNAL EAR

The most rapid period of growth and development of the human face takes place from the early part of the 4th week of embryonic life up to and including the 8th embryonic week[20] (Figs. 4, 5, 6). This phase, therefore, is a crucial period in the production of develop-

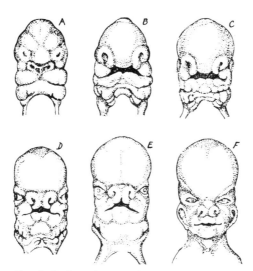

FIG. 4. Embryonic growth of the human face:
(*A*) 4-week embryo (3.5 mm); (*B*) 5-week embryo
(6.5 mm); (*C*) 6-week embryo (9 mm); (*D*) 6½-week
embryo (12 mm); (*E*) 7-week embryo (19 mm);
(*F*) 8-week embryo (28 mm) (after Patten). (From
Rogers, B. O., in *Reconstructive Plastic Surgery*, edited
by J. M. Converse, Vol. III, p. 1213. W. B. Saunders
Co., Philadelphia, 1964.)

mental aberrations. Since the Treacher-Collins syndrome and most craniofacial dysostoses are hereditary, one can naturally expect that the "pathologic" genes responsible for these facial malformations must play their principal role during this 4th to 8th week period.

Embryologically, the earliest signs of a "normal" definitive ear region appear as localized ectodermal thickenings. The otic placode, consisting of thickened ectodermal areas which presage the formation of the ear region, appears for the first time in embryos approximately 21 to 22 days old. Proliferation of the surrounding mesoderm then elevates the ectoderm around the edges of the placode so that the later soon takes on the appearance of an otic pit or otic depression, seen for the first time in the 26-day embryo (Fig. 5). By the 28th day, these pits become separated from the ectodermal surface, thus forming the otic vesicles (or otocysts).

As it elongates during the 5th embryonic week (29th–35th day), the oval otocyst in its more slender ventral portion shows signs of developing the future cochlear duct, whereas its more dorsal portions already indicate on the 34th day the site of the developing semicircular ducts and the intermediate positioned utricle and saccule. Primitive beginnings of the external ear, however, have not yet made their appearance until the very end of the 5th embryonic week.[22]

In the 39-day-old human embryo (12 mm), the right and left auricular regions occupy such a large surface area in their ventrolateral positions that there is only a very small interval of tissue between them from which the mandible and its associated soft parts will be derived (Fig. 6B). At this stage of embryologic development, therefore, the syndrome relationships which exist between some ear deformities and some mandibular deformities (see Figs. 18G, H, 19E, F), could be explained merely by the close physical proximity of these two regions and their susceptibility to the common action of any pathogen, genetic or otherwise.

Embryologic development is a fairly simple process to understand if one visualizes the growing mandible normally wedging the two auricles apart, as it begins to develop more rapidly in size than the neighboring external ear regions. In 33- and 39-day-old human embryos (Fig. 6A, B), the developing eye, ear, mandibular and maxillary areas lie so closely together that genetic or acquired factors leading to progressive damage or arrested growth in one of these loci might just as easily affect several or all of them at the same time. An example of this can be seen in patients with complete mandibulofacial dysostosis (Figs. 18F, 19C, D).

Despite these correlations between the physical proximity of some tissues and their common or

148

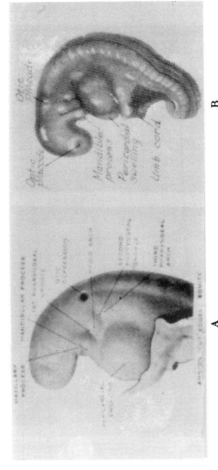

B

A

Fig. 5. (A) Lateral aspect of a 20-somite human embryo of approximately 26 days. (B) Left side of a 25-somite human embryo (3.4 mm) approximately 28 days old. (From Hamilton, W. J., Boyd, J. D., and Mossman, H. W.: *Human Embryology*, 3rd ed. The Williams and Wilkins Co., Baltimore, 1963.)

shared teratologic factors, such correlations have not been always remembered by surgeons or basic scientists, as these men studied or referred to the external ear and its malformations. Many clinicians, therefore, have referred erroneously to protruding, cup, and lop ears, as mere variations of "normal" ears, which project away from the mastoid area at exaggerated obtuse or right angles. In actuality, however, as in microtia, these ears represent true congenital deformities which can be traced to arrested stages of fetal development. In the young child, moreover, they give the clinician a clue as to the phase in intrauterine existence when the offending gene or genes responsible for the distorted shapes and sizes of these ears made its or their presence so strongly felt that no further developmental differentiation of the external ear into its "normal" adult form could take place.

There is no doubt that many protruding ears, cup ears, and lop ears are inherited. Genetic mechanisms are strongly implicated in their etiology, although there is also no doubt that some of these ears are the result of unknown environmental or "acquired" factors which retarded their final development into the normal ears which lie fairly close to the head in the newborn infant or young baby. Having inserted this brief departure from the narrative of embryologic development of the auricle, let us now return once again to the end of the 5th week of embryonic life and resume our story.

Normally the auricle develops around the first branchial groove, with tissue being supplied by both the first and second branchial arches (Fig. 6A). Initially in the 5-week-old embryo, (6 mm, 33 days) the mandibular and hyoid arches surrounding this first branchial groove have smooth margins (Fig. 6A). Soon, however, these margins begin to develop surface irregularities or hillocks which make their first appearance in the 11-mm (38-day-old) embryo (Fig. 6B). Three hillocks appear on the caudal border of the first arch and 3 can be seen during this period of development on the cephalic border of the second arch (Fig. 7A). By the end of the 6th embryonic week, on the 41st day, the 6 separate and distinct hillocks have begun to grow, have reached their maximum prominence, have moved

150

A   B

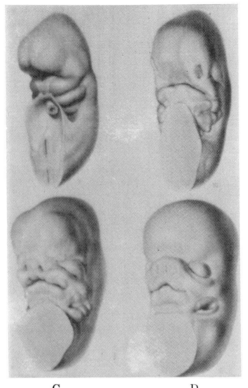

C   D

FIG. 6. Illustrations of ventrolateral views of the head in a series of human embryos, showing the change in topography of the auricle in the course of its development. (*A*) An embryo 6 mm long, 33 days old. The first and second branchial arches are very prominent, but smooth and free of hillocks. (*B*) An embryo 12 mm long, 39 days old. The auricular hillocks have appeared in the first and second branchial arches. (*C*) An embryo 14 mm long, 41 days old. The hillocks have begun to fuse and the *fossa angularis* has appeared. (*D*) An embryo 18 mm long, 45 days old. The hillock outlines are no longer observable, because fusion has almost been completed. (From Streeter, G. L.: Development of the auricle in the human embryo. Contrib. Embryol., Carnegie Inst., Washington, *14:* 111, 1922.)

from their initial ventral positions more dorsally and laterally, and have begun to fuse. By the 41st embryonic day, the 3 mandibular hillocks, which earlier covered most of the mandibular arch, now cover only its caudal margin. The 3 hyoid arch hillocks still occupy

151

the entire surface of the hyoid arch, except that portion which has become molded into the first branchial cleft or groove. At this 14-mm (41-day-old) stage, this cleft is much wider than in younger embryos and is a distinct entity, the *fossa angularis*. Deepening of the ventral third of this fossa now helps to form the primitive *external auditory meatus*, whereas the remaining mid- and dorsal two-thirds are eventually involved in formation of the auricle.

Some authors still believe that the supernumerary hillocks of His[23] are responsible for the small auricular appendages, especially the pre-auricular appendages frequently observed in front of the auricle (see Figs. 14F, I; 18B, C, G, H; 19E, F). His, in 1885 (Fig. 8), emphasized that the auricle develops in a rather precise manner from these 6 individual elevations and from an additional auricular fold of the hyoid integument.[23] He believed that hillock no. 1 formed the tragus (Fig. 8E), and that hillock no. 5 formed the antitragus. The remaining hillocks supposedly produced the rest of the auricle. One of the hillocks, possibly the third, was (and is still) thought by some authors to be responsible for Darwin's tubercle or the so-called "satyr" tip.

Schwalbe,[24] in 1897, also noted these 6 hillocks but he believed that the free helix margin of the external ear was derived not from them, but from a skin fold resembling an eyelid which appeared caudal to hillocks no. 4 and 5. This elevated, keel-like fold of skin remained as a protrusion until the 4th month, when it then became folded backwards in the region of the antihelix.[24] Thus, an incomplete folding caused persistence of the protruding ears in the post-natal infant. He suggested that anterior hillocks nos. 1, 2, and 3 were approximately identical in most persons, and that the external ears' physical individuality or specific characteristics were derived almost completely from the developing auricular fold.[25]

152

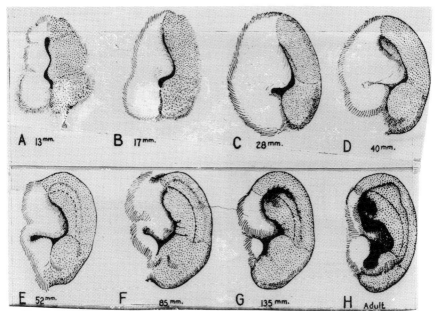

Fig. 7. *Part 1.* Stages in development of the external ear. The parts derived from the mandibular side of the cleft are unshaded; the parts from the hyoid side are indicated by stippling and by irregularly placed dashes. (After Streeter in Patten: *Human Embryology*, 2nd ed., McGraw-Hill Book Co., New York 1953.)

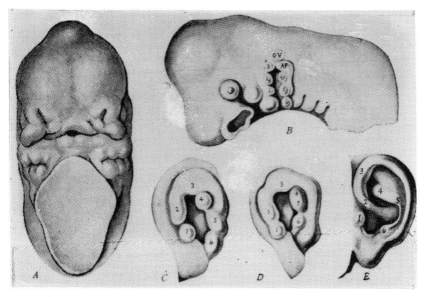

Fig. 8. *Part 2.* Development of the human auricle (partly after His). (*A*) Front view of the head, at 12.5 mm (× 13); below the face are the ear hillocks grouped about the first branchial grooves. (*B–E*) Side views of the auricle at 11 mm, 13.5 mm, 15 mm and in the adult. (*AF*, auricular fold; *OV*, otic vesicle; *1–6*, elevation on the mandibular and hyoid arches which respectively become: *1*, tragus; *2*, *3*, helix; *4*, *5*, antihelix; *6* antitragus. (From Arey: *Developmental Anatomy*, 6th ed. W. B. Saunders Co., Philadelphia 1954.)

153

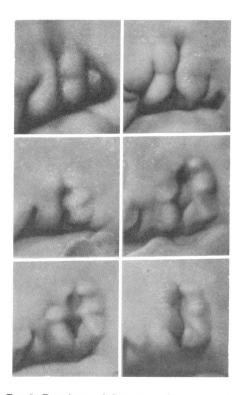

FIG. 9. Drawings of human embryos, showing the region of the first branchial cleft and its transformation into a fossa angularis. Coincident with this transformation the mesenchyme of the hyoid and mandibular bars undergoes proliferation and becomes condensed to form the primordium of the auricle. Foci of more active proliferation show on the surface as branchial hillocks. Specimens are from the Carnegie Collection.

    no. 13—5 mm long, 32 days old
    no. 14—11 mm long, 38 days old
    no. 15—10 mm long, 37 days old
    no. 16—13 mm long, 40 days old
    no. 17—14 mm long, 41 days old
    no. 18—15 mm long, 42 days old

(From Streeter, G. L.: Development of the auricle in the human embryo. Contrib. Embryol., Carnegie Inst. Washington, *14:* 111, 1922.)

Streeter[22] in 1922, however, restudied the entire embryology of the external ear in great detail, and disagreed with both His and Schwalbe. By examining many human embryos from the Carnegie collection (see Figs. 9–13), he concluded that the significance of

154

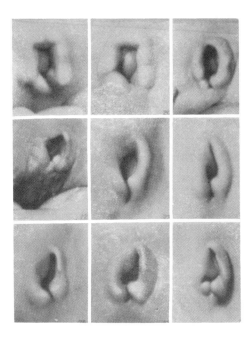

Fɪɢ. 10. Drawings of human embryos, in series
with the preceding plate (Figs. 9, nos. 13–18), and
showing the disappearance of the branchial hillocks
and the completion of the auricle in its primary form.
Specimens are from the Carnegie Collection.

no. 19—13 mm long, 40 days old
no. 20—15 mm long, 42 days old
no. 21—16.8 mm long, 43 days old
no. 22—17 mm long, 44 days old
no. 23—18 mm long, 45 days old
no. 24—17 mm long, 44 days old
no. 25—18 mm long, 45 days old
no. 26—21.3 mm long, 48 days old
no. 27—33.2 mm long, 59 days old

(From Streeter, G. L.: Development of the auricle
in the human embryo. Contrib. Embryol., Carnegie
Inst., Washington, *14:* 111, 1922.)

these hillocks or branchial arch tubercles had
been greatly over-emphasized, that they were
merely incidental and transitory rather than
serving as a fundamental factor in the development of the external ear. Streeter believed
that the external ear makes its first appearance embryologically as an intact primordium
that eventually grows and differentiates into
its final form, where it is "normally" positioned close to the side of the head and not

155

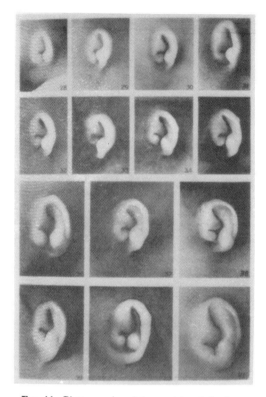

Fig. 11. Photographs of the auricle of the human fetus during the *third* month, all being taken at an enlargement of 10 diameters. In some cases the right ear was selected and reversed for convenience in comparison. These are indicated by the letter (R). All specimens are from the Carnegie Collection and length given is crown-rump.

no. 28—(28 mm)	no. 35—(50 mm)
no. 29—(36 mm)	no. 36—(52 mm) (R)
no. 30—(37 mm)	no. 37—(52 mm)
no. 31—(38.5 mm)	no. 38—(53 mm) (R)
no. 32—(40 mm) (R)	no. 39—(56.5 mm)
no. 33—(45.5 mm) (R)	no. 40—(57 mm)
no. 34—(49 mm)	no. 41—(62.5 mm) (R)

(From Streeter, G. L.: Development of the auricle in the human embryo. Contrib. Embryol., Carnegie Inst., Washington, *14:* 111, 1922).

protruding from it.

This primordium makes itself evident microscopically as a distinct ectodermal mesenchymal activity, the ectoderm actually serving as a mirror of the primitive cartilaginous form of the ear. This ectodermal activity is accompanied by marked prolifera-

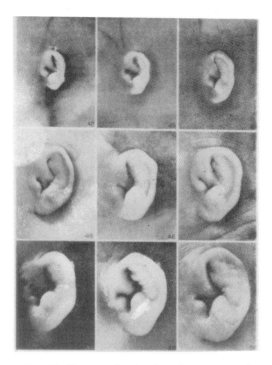

FIG. 12. Photographs showing changes occurring in the auricle of the human fetus during the *fourth* month. In some cases the right ear was selected and reversed for convenience in comparison. These are indicated by the letter (R). All the photographs are taken at an enlargement of 6 diameters. Specimens are from the Carnegie Collection, and length given is crown-rump.

no. 42—(66.2 mm)	no. 47—(87.3 mm)
no. 43—(65 mm)	no. 48—(103.5 mm)
no. 44—(69 mm)	no. 49—(100 mm) (R)
no. 45—(85 mm)	no. 50—(113 mm) (R)
no. 46—(87 mm)	

(From Streeter, G. L.: Development of the auricle in the human embryo. Contrib. Embryol., Carnegie Inst., Washington, *14:* 111, 1922).

tion and condensation of the mesenchyme in the juxtaposed portions of the first and second branchial arches. The hillocks, therefore, are merely foci of mesenchymal proliferation, and they have largely smoothed out at the 16–18 mm stage (43rd–45th day) (Fig. 10 nos. 21–23), with the exception of those which continue as the antitragus and tragus (Fig. 7B—17 mm). Soon thereafter a specific layer of

157

pre-cartilage cells can be seen which essentially resembles the shape of the adult cartilage of the future pinna. According to Streeter, the antihelix is formed beneath the smooth external ear surface very early in the 16–18 mm (43rd–44th day or 2nd month) and is not the product of a much later backward folding or compression, as suggested by Schwalbe. Streeter admitted that some of his older fetal ears have a "poorly marked helix," e.g., lopping (Fig. 13, nos. 51–54), which by persisting into the 5th month indicated that not every ear in his study was truly "normal."

In the 44-day embryo, the fused hillocks completely surround the developing external auditory meatus which represents the persisting ventral portion of the first pharyngeal groove (see Fig. 7B—17 mm).

Whereas during the 6th week this developing ear region first appeared in a ventromedial position, with gradual growth of the face and the lower jaw during the 7th week this primitive pinna continues to become displaced more dorsolaterally (Fig. 4D–F).

In the 13–17 mm stage (Fig. 7A, B), which corresponds roughly to the 40–44 day of embryologic development, the amount of mandibular and hyoid mesenchyme which forms the external ear seems to be roughly equal, but during the later phase of the 7th and 8th weeks of embryologic development, and subsequently during fetal development of the ear, the amount of mandibular arch mesenchyme gradually decreases at the expense of the hyoid arch mesenchyme. The latter, therefore, eventually contributes to the formation of 85 per cent or more of the adult external ear (Fig. 7H).

The only portions of the ear eventually derived from the mandibular arch are the anterior crus of the helix margin and the tragus. The hyoid arch contributes the helix, antihelix, scapha, antitragus, and the lobule.

158

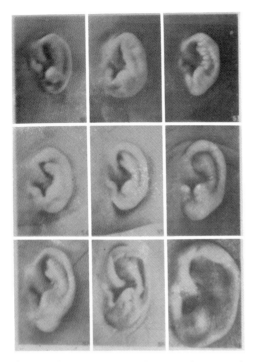

FIG. 13. Photographs showing the form of the human auricle during the *fifth* month of intrauterine life, with the exception of specimen shown in no. 59, which has a menstrual age of 23 weeks. The photographs are all shown at an enlargement of 4 diameters. Specimens are from the Carnegie Collection, and length given is crown-rump.

no. 51—(113.5 mm)	no. 56—(135.6 mm)
no. 52—(114 mm)	no. 57—(150 mm)
no. 53—(114 mm)	no. 58—(154 mm)
no. 54—(119 mm)	no. 59—(191.2 mm)
no. 55—(119 mm)	

(From Streeter, G. L.: Development of the auricle in the human embryo, Contrib. Embryol., Carnegie Inst., Washington, *14:* 111, 1922).

The cleft lying between the first and second branchial arch has become the fossa angularis. The tissues lying in the floor of this cleft eventually form the head of Meckel's cartilage. The very last portion of the external ear to make its appearance is the concha; the tragus, which intially existed as a two-lobed structure, sometimes persists in that form in certain individuals. The persistence of other

159

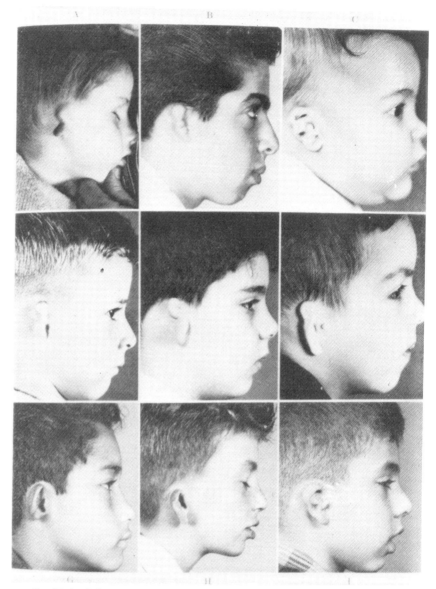

FIG. 14. (*A–I*) Cases of microtia in a sequence of decreasing severity, gradually advancing into the stage of "lop" ear deformity, in which the lop ear is usually smaller than a "normal" ear and is characterized by a curling forward and downward of the upper pole of the ear, often with a marked shortage of skin coverage in this region (see Figs. 15.4–*F*).

A. Very severe microtia.

B. Posterior margins of microtic remnant suggestive of persistence of embryonic hillocks.

C. Anterior and posterior margins of this crumpled microtic ear suggest persistence of 6 embryonic hillocks.

D and E. Lobule more developed than upper pole.

F. Microtic remnant with pre-auricular appendage.

G. Small microtic ear with deficient lobule.

H. Small microtic ear with deficient upper pole.

I. Small microtic "lop" ear with pre-auricular appendage.

160

"embryologic-fetal arrests" of normal development into adult life, combined with certain features of auricular abnormal development, will now be dealt with in more detail.

"CIRCUMSTANTIAL" POST-NATAL EVIDENCE OF EMBRYOLOGIC-FETAL MALDEVELOPMENT

A study of hundreds of clinical photographs of ear deformities (Figs. 14–22) gave me the impression that I was observing almost every conceivable type of congenital ear deformity that any comparable large plastic surgery clinic would be confronted with in a 20-year period. As such, these photographs could be considered as post-natal circumstantial evidence of embryologic-fetal development or maldevelopment—"circumstantial" in that as post-natal material they could probably be arranged in a logical photographic sequence providing the viewer with a glimpse into embryologic-fetal events (without the need for examining actual human embryos, the supply of which is certainly rare under most conditions).

It has been my contention for several years[20] that there is considerable overlapping of the physical characteristics of many forms of microtia, lop, cup, and protruding ears. I will attempt in these photographs (Figs. 14–17) to correlate our post-natal clinical examples of these external ear deformities with the majority of Streeter's illustrations and photographs of embryologic and fetal development of the external ear (Figs. 6–7 and 9–13). The use of sequential photographic material in this manner, therefore, might permit an investigator to make deductions from "post-facto" evidence, when "de-facto" evidence in human embryos is scarce or lacking.

We must ask ourselves, however, if it is logical or acceptable to arrange this *post-facto* evidence in an orderly sequence. If it is, the developmental events of embryonic life could be inferred from the phenotypic or post-natal expressions of an

161

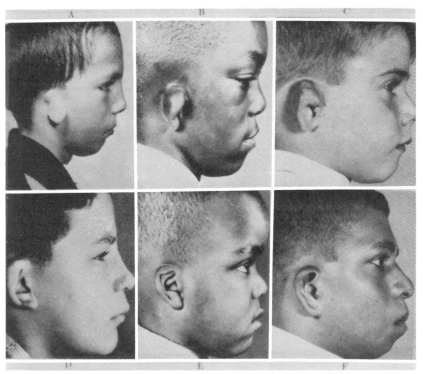

FIG. 15. (A–E) Lop ears characterized in a sequence of decreasing severity, terminating in a cup ear deformity (F).

A. Severe microtia–lop ear, in which the upper pole of the ear has dropped over the intact lobule—a truly limp or lop ear.
B. Severe lopping of upper pole of ear.
C. Severe lopping of upper pole, with deficient skin coverage.
D. Less severe lop ear.
E. Only margin of upper pole of ear is flattened and deficient.
F. Lop ear merging in its characteristics with a cup ear.

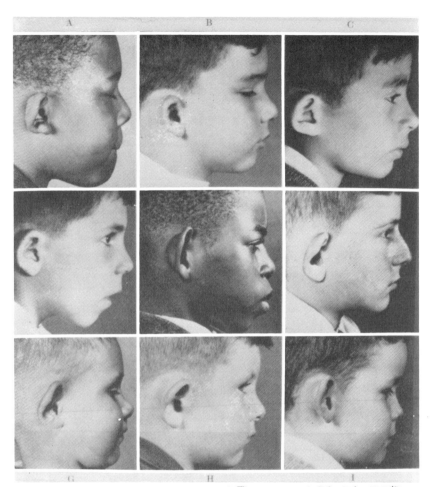

FIG. 16. (A–I) Severely protruding cup ears (A–E) in a sequence of decreasing severity, terminating in or merging with more typical protruding ear (F–I) deformities. Most cup ears are smaller than protruding ears. (E) Observe the extreme conchal overdevelopment and protrusion which contributes to the cupping.

163

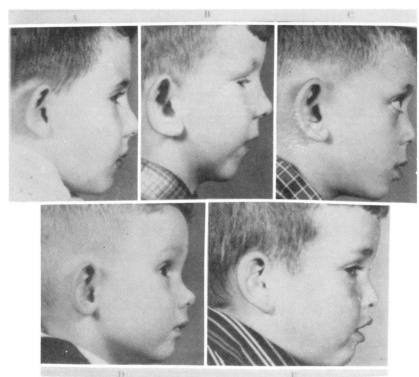

Fig. 17. (A–E) Protruding ears in a sequence of decreasing severity, terminating in a "normal" ear (E) with its flatter shape and positioned closer to the head and mastoid process.

anomaly. Assuming that this indirect investigational approach is used systematically, one could hope to learn from this approach.

In the motion picture film shown with this paper, it was possible by dissolve-action photography to blend or "dissolve" from one photograph into another, thus giving the viewer the illusion of observing a phase–by–phase development, or maldevelopment, of the external ear as it probably occurs in the embryo and fetus.

As this motion picture film can not be reproduced on the printed page, the following still photographs (Figs. 14–17 and 20–22) have been arranged to give the reader a similar (but not quite as satisfactory) visual experience, in so far as that is possible. This is a highly controversial method of describing embryologic and fetal development, of course, but it is hopefully offered to stimulate new thought about methods which experimental embryologists and teratologists might possibly use to study post-natal material as a guide to embryonic and fetal growth, development, and maldevelopment.

If this method proves to be valid, one might employ it to better our understanding of the sequential maldevelopments in such deformities as cleft lip, micrognathia, colobomata, hypertelorism, bifid nose, microphthalmos, etc.

Certainly the similarities between many of our clinical photographs and Streeter's human embryo ears (Figs. 9–13) would seem to be more than mere happenstance. For example, by comparing the 17-mm human embryo ear in Figure 10, no. 24 with the microtic ear remnant in Figure 14D, one might assume or state that the child's microtic ear had never developed beyond the 17-mm stage (the 44th day or early in the 7th week of embryologic development; see Table 32-1 in Rogers[20]).

If, however, a microtic ear is slightly more differentiated in its development (Fig. 14G), one might similarly or "circumstantially" state that this ear had never developed beyond the 33.2-mm stage (the 58–59th day, or early in the 9th week of fetal development; see Fig. 10, no. 27).

It soon becomes apparent by comparatively examining the embryologic and clinical illustrations and photographs (Figs. 8, 9, nos. 13–18, 10, nos. 19–26, 14A–F, 18F–H, 19A–D, and 20A–E) that the most severe forms of microtia typified only by very small ear

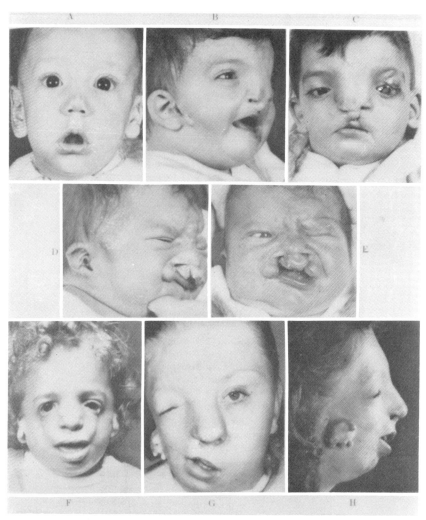

Fig. 18. (A–H) Cases of ear deformities with other gross craniofacial abnormalities or stigmata. (A) Left microtia, lop ear deformity; slight nasal tip bifidity, perhaps representing a "forme fruste" of the disorder seen in B and C. (B and C) Absent right and left tragus, hypertelorism, bifid nose, colobomata, bilateral cleft lip, cleft palate, congenital cataracts. (D and E) Bilateral microtia with absent lobules, bilateral cleft lip, and cleft palate. (F) Severe mandibulofacial dysostosis including bilateral microtia, lop ear deformity, a malar hypoplasia, colobomata, deafness, etc. (c.f. Rogers[21]). (G and H) Severe unilateral first and second branchial arch syndrome with persistence of embryonic hillocks in their more ventral and medial embryonal position, misplaced in this patient's cheek region.

166

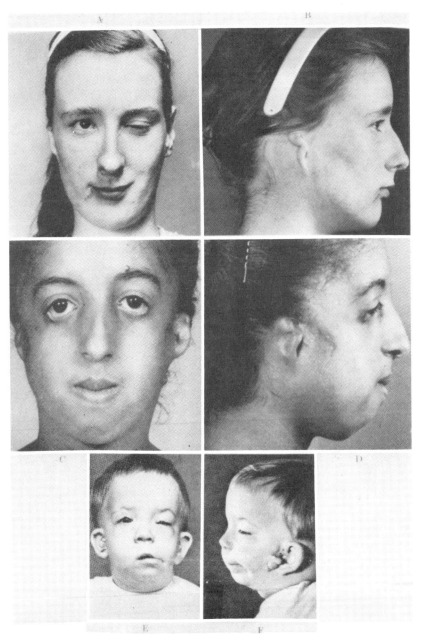

FIG. 19. (A–F) Cases of ear deformities with other gross craniofacial abnormalities. (A and B) Unilateral right microtia with right facial paralysis. (C and D) Bilateral microtia in a case of mandibulofacial dysostosis (c.f. Rogers[21]). (E and F) Bilateral pre-auricular appendages and absent tragus in lop–cup ear deformities, with macrostomia, left hemignathia, and colobomata.

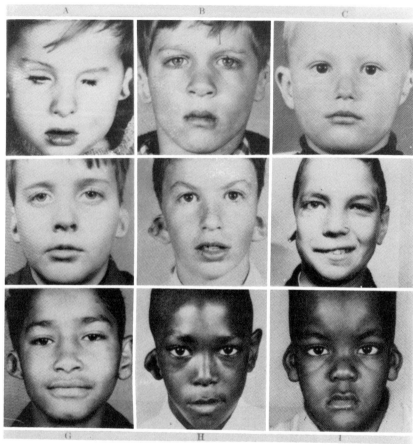

FIG. 20. (A–I) Cases of ear deformities in a sequence of decreasing severity, ranging from severe bilateral microtia (A, B, D) to microtia–lop ear deformities (F–I).

A. Microphthalmos and facial asymmetry present.

D and E. Deficient upper poles of the ears bilaterally.

F. Severe, limp lopping of the microtic upper pole, which covers an intact lobule.

I. Deficient skin coverage in the margins of the lopped upper pole.

"remnants" largely represent arrests in *embryologic development* (6th–8th weeks, 10 mm–33.2 mm), whereas the more minor degrees of microtia reflect some disturbance in *fetal development* of the ear region 3rd month, 31–62.5 mm; see Figs. 10, no. 27, 11, nos. 28–41, 14*G–I*, 20*F–I*, 21*A–E*).

These photographic sequences also suggest that there might be a later or more mature stage in fetal development during which the auricle continues to develop along fairly normal patterns until it is arrested at a later protruding phase of development (see fetal ear in Fig. 12, nos. 42–44). Or it may develop less completely along partially "microtic" patterns, in which case the arrested result is a lop ear, usually smaller than a normal ear, typified by a downward acute folding of the scapha and helix at about the tuberculum auriculae level in association with faulty development of the antihelix (see fetal ears in Fig. 11, nos. 31–41). The lop ear, therefore, usually has features of its preceding embryonic microtic stage; it represents, in the normal sequence of development or maldevelopment, a stage lying between microtia and protrusion. Similarly, the cup ear is probably another stage of development or maldevelopment, which also lies between microtia and protrusion, but it is at a more mature stage in its development only because of the late appearance of the developing concha; thus, it has characteristics more typical of the protruding ear than of the microtic ear.

McEvitt,[26] in 1947, was one of the first to summarize the developmental inter-relationships between protruding ears and other true ear deformities, as follows: "Protrusion may be unilateral or bilateral. It may be associated with other congenital deformities such as reduplicated Darwinian tubercle, absence of the lobule, microtia of any degree, macrotia, curling, or displacement. It is sometimes seen in association with marked facial asym-

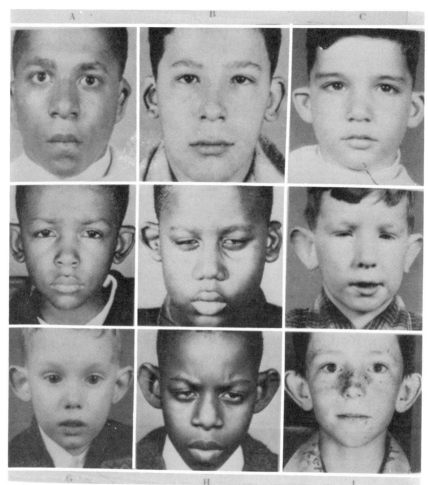

Fig. 21. (A–I) Cases of ear deformities in a sequence of decreasing severity, ranging from lop–cup ears (A–E) to more truly cup ears (F–H) and finally to protruding ears (I).

metry." Others since McEvitt, including Holmes[27] in 1949, Stephenson[28] in 1960, and Musgrave[29] in 1966, have also drawn attention to these inter-relationships of ear deformities.

There is no doubt that lop ears, cup ears, and protruding ears share one feature in common which is not found in the fully developed normal adult ear, namely—a faulty or incomplete development of the antihelix. Perhaps more emphasis should be placed upon the word "incomplete" rather than "faulty," a word which Streeter also found preferable. It is of more than passing interest that in Wildervanck's study,[19] regardless of the type of ear deformity inherited by the first and second generation of children in the family studied, all deformities shown in the photographs in his report (and these included cases of microtia with a crumpled upper pole, lop ears with a flattened superior margin of the helix and flattened antihelix, low implantation of small lop and cup ears, and typical protruding ears of normal size), all were characterized by an incomplete development of the antihelix and the helix' superior margin. Wildervanck's study, therefore, seems to support the concept stressed in this paper that the developing ear advances through a sequence of morphologic changes which begin with "microtia"-like phases—and then it progresses through the phases of "lopping," "cupping," and "protruding," before finally terminating in the flattened, normal, adult ear with its well-developed (or completely developed) antihelix and a not overly developed conchal region.

GENETIC COUNSELING

Of what significance are these findings, especially those stressing the inheritance of these deformities, for the plastic surgeon, geneticist, or teratologist? One answer to this question lies in the field of genetic counseling.

171

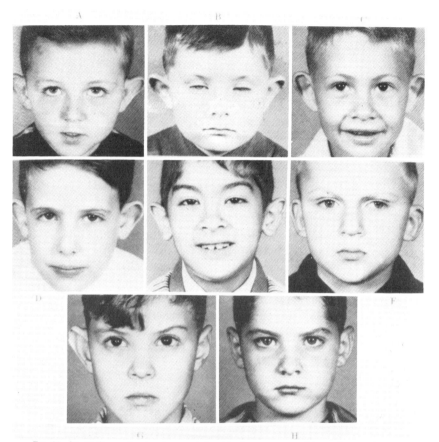

FIG. 22. (A–H) Cases of protruding ear deformities in a sequence of decreasing severity with the ears gradually assuming their more "normal" flattened position, closer to the head (H).

172

It is best summarized by Wildervanck, as follows:

"The two families I visited ... asked me, of course, about the future progeny of their affected children. If there is a full penetration of the gene— and this seems to be so, as ten children of the three affected brothers show an aberration, and eleven are normal, which we may expect in a dominant mode of heredity with full penetration—we are justified in telling the parents that each child of their affected children has a 50% chance of showing the syndrome in a mild or severe form. A child severely affected [ed: with microtia or lop or cup ears] ... may get children who show deafness or microtia; it is, however, also possible that they will only show a ... [protruding] ... ear, pit or appendage. The future children of boys and girls who are only slightly affected stand the same chance. These children may show a pit, but a severe conductive deafness is possible too! The fact that the first father, who only shows one ... [lop and one protruding ear] ... got two children who are severely handicapped, makes the latter point clear. But, as only two of the 14 abnormal members of the family are severely affected, the chance that they may show only a ... [lop or protruding ear], an appendage or a pit, is much greater." [19]

In essence, Wildervanck's summary suggests that in any single family in which both the mother and father are afflicted with one of these 4 disorders and/or pre-auricular or auricular pits, fistulae, or appendages, genetic counseling should definitely be considered because of the high degree of likelihood that offspring born to these parents will be simi-larly afflicted, quite often with a more severe form of the disorder.

SUMMARY

An attempt is made to show the embryo-logic-fetal development of the external ear as it might take place, based upon the use of multiple, still photographs of clinical ear deformities, arranged in a photographic sequence to give the reader a *post-facto* record of embryonic-fetal development of the auricle.

These still photographs were originally

173

presented in a motion picture, with "dissolve" action photography to blend or dissolve from one photograph into the other. These gave the viewer the illusion of observing phase-by-phase development, or maldevelopment, of the external ear as it probably occurs in the embryo and fetus. It is hoped that this technique of sequential photographic studies of a surface anomaly may prove to be helpful to plastic surgeons and teratologists alike in studying other craniofacial anomalies, such as cleft lip, bifid nose, hypertelorism, and colobomata.

The report has attempted to show, also, the morphologic, anatomical, and genetic interrelationships that exist between microtia, lop ears, cup ears, and protruding ears, all of which are inherited in a large number of instances. An attempt to differentiate between, and to correlate, the morphologic and anatomical characteristics of microtic ears, lop ears, cup ears, and protruding ears has been made. From the available evidence, it seems that there are strong inheritable genetic factors active in the etiology of these 4 inter-related deformities. The appearance of one or another of these ear abnormalities, or of combinations of them, may merely be the result of the variable expression of, and the strength or weakness of the degree of penetrance of the offending genes.

Thus, in any single family in which both the mother and father are afflicted with 1 of these 4 disorders (and/or pre-auricular or auricular pits, fistulae, or appendages) genetic counseling should be considered because of the likelihood that offspring born to these parents will be similarly afflicted—quite often with a more severe form of the disorder.

Supported in part by a grant from the Association for the Aid of Crippled Children, New York, N. Y.

ACKNOWLEDGMENT

The author is deeply grateful to Dr. John Marquis Converse for his helpful suggestions and encouragement of this study.

REFERENCES

1. Heywoode, J.: *John Heywoodes Workes . . . Proverbes . . .* Part I, Ch. VIII, 1598. Cited in *Familiar Quotations by John Bartlett*, 13th ed., p. 94a. Little Brown and Co., Boston, 1955.
2. Johnson, T.: *The Works of that Famous Chirurgeon Ambrose Parey, Translated out of Latin and Compared with the French by Th. Johnston:* Printed by Mary Clark, and are to be sold by John Clark, at Mercers Chappel, at the Lower End of Cheapside, London, p. 126, 1678.
3. Davis, J. S.: *Plastic Surgery: Its Principles and Practice,* p. 425. P. Blakiston's Son & Co., Philadelphia, 1919.
4. Swift, J.: *To Dr. Delany,* 1729. Cited in *A New Dictionary of Quotations on Historical Principles from Ancient and Modern Sources,* selected and edited by H. L. Mencken, p. 326. Alfred A. Knopf, New York, 1960.
5. Hopkins, G. M.: *The Habit of Perfection.* Cited in *Familiar Quotations by John Bartlett*, 13th ed. p. 724b. Little Brown and Co., Boston, 1955.
6. Coon, C. S., and Hunt, E. E., Jr.: *The Living Races of Man,* pp. 12, 113, 124. Alfred A. Knopf, New York, 1965.
7. Hooton, E. A.: *Crime and the Man,* pp. 126–127, 269, 275. Harvard University Press, Cambridge, Mass., 1939.
8. Coon, C. S., and Hunt, E. E., Jr. (editors).: *Anthropology A to Z,* p. 200. Universal Reference Library. Grosset & Dunlap, Inc., New York, 1963.
9. Montagu, A.: *Human Heredity,* p. 223. A Mentor Book. The New American Library of World Literature, Inc., New York, 1960.
10. Winchester, A. M.: *Heredity and Your Life,* 2nd ed., p. 317. Dover Publications, Inc., New York, 1960.
11. Siemens, H. W.: Zur Kenntnis der sogenannten Ohr-und Halsanhänge (branchiogene Knorpelnaevi). Arch. Dermat. u. Syph., *132:* 186, 1921.
12. Kindred, J. E.: Inheritance of a pit in the skin of the left ear. J. Hered., *12:* 366, 1921.

13. Quelprud, T.: Ear pit and its inheritance. J. Hered., *31:* 379, 1940.
14. Ruttin, E.: Zur Frage der Fistula auris congenita und der Aurikularanhänge. Wien. med. Wchnschr., *77:* 1019, 1927.
15. Powell, E. F., and Whitney, D. D.: Ear lobe inheritance: an unusual three-generation photographic pedigree-chart. J. Hered., *28:* 185, 1937.
16. Potter, E. L.: A hereditary ear malformation: transmitted through five generations. J. Hered., *28:* 255, 1937.
17. Brander, T.: Zur Kenntnis der Ätiologie der Ohranhänge. Acta dermat.-venereol., *20:* 213, 1939.
18. Hanhart, E.: Nachweis einer einfach-dominanten, unkomplizierten sowie unregelmässig-. dominanten, mit *Atresia auris, Palatoschisis* und anderen Deformationen verbundenen Anlage zu Ohrmuschelverkümmerung (Mikrotie). Arch. Julius Klaus-Stift., *24:* 374, 1949.
19. Wildervanck, L. S.: Hereditary malformations of the ear in three generations: marginal pits, pre-auricular appendages, malformations of the auricle and conductive deafness. Acta oto-laryng., *54:* 553, 1962.
20. Rogers, B. O.: Chapter 32: Rare craniofacial deformities. In *Reconstructive Plastic Surgery,* edited by J. M. Converse, Vol. III, Ch. 32, p. 1213. W. B. Saunders Co., Philadelphia, 1964.
21. Rogers, B. O.: Berry-Treacher Collins syndrome: a review of 200 cases. Brit. J. Plast. Surg., *17:* 109, 1964.
22. Streeter, G. L.: Development of the auricle in the human embryo. Contrib. Embryol., Carnegie Inst., Washington, *14:* 111, 1922.
23. His, W.: Die Formentwicklung des ausseren Ohres. In *Anatomie menschlicher Embryonen,* Part III, p. 211. F. C. W. Vogel, Leipzig, 1885.
24. Schwalbe, G.: Das äussere Ohr. In *Handbuch der Anatomie des Menschen,* by K. von Bardeleben, Vol. 5, part 2, pp. 125–131, 1897.
25. Stark, R. B., and Saunders, D. E.: Natural appearance restored to the unduly prominent ear. Brit. J. Plast. Surg., *15:* 385, 1962.
26. McEvitt, W. G.: The problem of the protruding ear. Plast. & Reconstr. Surg., *2:* 481, 1947.
27. Holmes, E. M.: The microtic ear. Arch. Otol., *49:* 243, 1949.
28. Stephenson, K. L.: Correction of a lop ear type deformity. Plast. & Reconstr. Surg., *26:* 540, 1960.
29. Musgrave, R. H.: A variation on the correction of the congenital lop ear. Plast. & Reconstr. Surg., *37:* 394, 1966.
30. Ely, E. T.: An operation for prominence of the auricles. Arch. Otol., *10:* 97, 1881.

EXPERIENCES FROM 5 YEARS OF GENETIC COUNSELING IN EYE DISEASES

By

Ernst Goldschmidt

In the 5-year period from 1st January 1961 to 1st January 1966 2932 coun-seling cases were dealt with at the University Institute of Human Genetics, Copenhagen. A total of 185 cases (4.7 per cent) are concerned with eye dis-eases and Table 1 gives a survey of the reasons for referring these cases to the Institute. About two-thirds come from *Mødrehjælpen* (Mothers Aid Cen-tres), which, apart from dealing with applications for legal abortion and sterilization also mediate in cases of adoption. In the latter instance, ap-plication is made to the Institute in order to ascertain whether the child to be adopted will be liable to suffer from a serious hereditary disease that would make adoption inadvisable. These cases are but few. Most of the cases concern requests for legal abortion, and in the declaration made by the In-stitute an estimate is given of the presumed risk of an hereditary lesion in the expected baby, but it does not state whether such risk should consitute an eugenic indication for legal abortion. This can only be decided upon by the joint council of the Mothers Aid Centres. It is our impression that the

Table 1

185 counseling cases classified according to reasons for being referred to the Institute of Human Genetics.

	Number of cases
Adoption	8
Legal abortion	81
Sterilization	10
Legal Abortion + Sterilization	22
Eugenic counseling	42
Registration	22
Total	185

177

Pregnancy Act is interpreted in such a way that when the risk of a serious lesion is 10 % or more, legal abortion on eugenic grounds is indicated.

Forty-two of the cases deal with advice to young people who are considering marriage, or to parents who have had a child with an eye lesion that could be genetically determined. More than half this group come from the State Institute for the Blind, where Chief Physician *H. Skydsgaard,* has for many years considered it of the utmost significance to give his pupils eugenic instruction and advice before they finish their training. (cf. *Skydsgaard* (1957)). The advice given is based on a declaration from the Institute. This, in my opinion, is the best procedure , since the adviser ought to be a doctor with intimate knowledge of the patient as well as of his or her eventual partner.

The last group comprises partly registration of families with an hereditary eye lesion, partly enquiries as to whether the Institute has any information on a given family.

Table 2 gives a survey of the most frequently occurring diagnoses. Naturally, a material of this nature does not offer any information as to the incidence of the various eye lesions among the population, but it does give an idea of the relative frequency. It is, however, probable that eye lesions such as have been the subject of more detailed anlysis in a recent Danish thesis, for in-

Table 2

Ocular anomalies in 185 counseling cases.

Disorders of the eyeball

Anophthalmos	4
Microphthalmos	4
Colobomata	10
Aniridia	9
Ectopia lentis	8
Congenital glaucoma	8
Glaucoma simplex	1
Myopia excessiva	18

Anomalies of motility and eyelids

Ptosis	1
Strabismus	1
Nystagmus	3
Blepharophimosis	1

Anomalies of pigmentation

Ocular albinism	2

Corneal dystrophy 1

Congenital cataract 39

Anomalies of the retina

Achromatopsia	2
Tapeto-retinal degenerations	30

Optic atrophy

Leber's disease	3
Infantile dominant atrophy	5
Unknown etiology	5

Tumors and pseudotumors

Retinoblastoma	6
Norrie's disease	6
Retrolental fibroplasia	2

Phakomatoses 7

Lipoidoses 7

Cranio-facial dysostoses 5

Table 3

Survey of 39 cases of congenital cataract.

Familial cases

 Dominant mode of inheritance 14
 Recessive mode of inheritance 2

Sporadic cases

 Rubella embryopathy 3
 Unknown etiology 17

Secondary cases

 Lowe's syndrome 1
 With aniridia 1
 With ectopia lentis 1

stance, infantile dominant optic atrophy (*Kjer* (1959) and Norrie's disease (*Warburg* (1967)), will occur somewhat more freqently because the members of the known families have been informed of the eugenic problems during their contact with the ophthalmologist.

The group: Colobomata mostly comprises cases of coloboma of the iris but also a few of the chorioid.

In the group: ectopia lentis there are 3 patients with luxation of the lens without any other symptoms, 4 cases of Marfan's syndrome, and one case of associated ectopia of the lens and pupil.

In the group of excessive myopias several families with retinal detachment are recorded.

The retinal degenerations constitute quite a large group in which typical retinopathia pigmentosa occurs the most frequently. Out of 15 families the mode of inheritance was recessive in 11, dominant in 2, sex-linked revessive in 1, and possibly irregularly dominant in 1. In 2 of the recessive families the patients were also deaf.

This group further includes cases of Laurence-Moon-Biedl's syndrome, Leber's infantile amaurosis, and a few cases that could not be classified with certainty.

Out of 13 cases of optic atrophy, 5 were of the infantile dominant type, 3 patients had Leber's disease and in 5 cases the etiology was obscure.

By far the most frequently occurring lesion is congenital cataract (Table 3). In Denmark we have several large cataract families with typical dominant mode of inheritance. One of these families has been followed through 9 generations and was last reported by *Marner* in 1950. Among 39 cases, 4 are related to this family, and in altogether 16 cases several family members have cataract.

20 cataract cases occur sporadically, and the etiology is only known in a

very few cases. Thus, 3 are presumably caused by rubella embryopathy, while as far as could be ascertained from the information received, none of them were due to radiation during pregnancy. Some of the sporadic cataracts may be genetic mutations, but we do not know the mutation rate, nor the frequency of environmentally determined congenital cataracts. Neither is there any mention in the literature of an empiric risk figure for the offspring of sporadic cataracts. In these cases we have given patients who apply for legal abortion the benefit of the doubt, and have informed the Mothers Aid Centres that it cannot be excluded that the risk of congenital cataract in children of "sporadic" parents is very great (up to 50 %). It is, however, far more difficult to give advice to parents who wish to have children. In this connection it must be realised that recessive forms of congenital cataract do exist—and that their prognosis usually is poor. I have two failies in which this mode of inheritance is probable. In one of them there are 3 sibs with cataract and nystagmus, all of whom are at the State Institute for the Blind.

In the material there are 3 families in which, apart from cataract, deafness occurs at the adult age. I have not seen this condition mentioned in the literature.

In Table 4 I have collected cases in which both parents are blind in an attempt to ascertain whether a poorer eugenic prognosis might result from the fact that young blind persons gather at special institutions while they are being trained.

In dominant traits the choice of the partner is of no particular significance

Table 4

Ocular anomalies in 14 blind or weak-sighted parents.

Diagnoses.

No.	Father	Mother
1	Buphthalmos	Congenital cataract + nystagmus
2	Buphthalmos	Buphthalmos
3	Buphthalmos	Buphthalmos
4	Buphthalmos	Microphthalmos + coloboma iridis
5	Congenital cataract	Retinopathia pigmentosa
6	Congenital cataract	Myopia excessiva
7	Congenital cataract	Myopia excessiva
8	Chorioiditidis seq.	Myopia excessiva
9	Coloboma nn. optici	Congenital cataract + microphthalmos
10	Microphthalmos dxt.	Aniridia
11	Myopia excessiva	Myopia excessiva + colob. macul. dxt.
12	Nystagmus cong.	Aniridia
13	Retinopathia pigmentosa	Aniridia
14	Tapeto-retinal degeneration (uncertain type)	Congenital cataract

to the prognosis, but in recessive traits it is obvious that the choice of partner is of the utmost importance. If the partner is chosen who is not related to the patient, and in whose family the same trait is not recorded, the risk is generally less than 1 %, since most of the more serious recessive lesions occur with a frequency around 1 in 10000. If, on the other hand, a partner with the same lesion is chosen, then all the children born of those parents will be affected.

From the table it will be seen that practically only in families 2 and 3 is the choice of the partner unfavorable from an eugenic point of view.

In the first family the mother has 2 sisters, both of whom are blind, one of them also with buphthalmia. The other sister is in the care of the Danish Service for the Mentally Retarded, but is living with a private family. She probably has buphthalmia, too. There are no other known cases of buphthalmia in the father's family. This couple has two children. Shortly after birth the older child was admitted to an Eye Department, where bilateral aniridia was diagnosed. The second child was born in 1961 and, according to information from the parents to the Mothers Aid Centre, the child has normal vision.

In the other family the mother's sister also has buphthalmia. There are no other cases in the father's family. In 1960 they had a child who since birth has a rather large cornea measuring over 13 mm in diameter, but that otherwise the cornea is quite normal. The child's sight is normal, tension normal, gonioscopy and ophthalmoscopy normal. Later the mother had a legal abortion on eugenic indication, and has been sterilized.

I have mentioned these two families partly because nothing has even been published about children whose parents both had buphthalmia, partly in order to demontrate that things do not always happen just as the books say. It is hardly correct that buphthalmia is always inherited. Phenocopies are also seen, in line with what we see in congenital cataract, retinoblastoma, and excessive myopia.

For genetic counseling purposes it is evident that the complete medical history of the case has to be obtained and more knowledge is often required than for a clinical diagnosis. Unfortunately such non-classifiable diagnoses as uveitis foetalis, congenital amaurosis, and retinal degenerations are not infrequently met with and ophthalmologists should not hesitate in examining children in anaesthesia, take ERG etc. to ensure a clear diagnosis.

Even if a case looks quite clear a simple collection of information about both parents and their families should never be omitted. The minimum requirement includes a search for any significant deviations from the normal in the parents, the sibs, the sibs of the parents and the grandparents of the child, and in some cases this is not enough. All information obtained from the patients or their parents should be verified and supplemented by con-

181

tacts with hospitals and other medical services in order to establish the most precise genetic information.

It is the task of the ophthalmologist to prevent blindness, and it is consequently a part of his work to draw attention to the risk of giving birth to blind children, when such a risk is present. It is, however, not his task to take any decision on behalf of those who come for counseling but only to assist them in finding their own solution to the problems. Genetic counseling is familial guidance and should not be based on considerations of a socio-economic nature but be regarded as one of the tools of preventive medicine.

References

Kjer, P.: Infantile optic atrophy with dominant mode of inheritance. Copenhagen 1959.
Marner, E.: A family with eight generations of hereditary cataract. *Acta Ophthal.* (Kbh.) 1949, 27 : 537.
Skydsgaard, H.: On eugenic problems in the prevention of blindness. *Acta Ophthal.* (Kbh.) 1957, 35 : 325.
Warburg, M.: Norrie's Disease. *Acta Ophthal.* (Kbh.) Supplementum 89, 1966.

X-linked Hydrocephalus

MICHAEL W. SHANNON and HENRY L. NADLER

Since the original description of a sex-linked mode of inheritance in congenital hydrocephalus (Bickers and Adams, 1949), subsequent reports have been published presenting additional families in which this inheritance pattern appeared to be present. Bamatter (1949) described a family in which the mother had delivered 2 hydrocephalic males and 3 normal females. Zimmer (1952) reviewed a family with 3 stillborn hydrocephalic males, while Borle (1953) reported 3 hydrocephalic brothers in one family. Gellman (1959) presented twin hydrocephalic brothers. Edwards, Norman, and Roberts (1961) and Edwards (1961), described 4 families with histories of hydrocephalus, one with 15 affected males. Needleman and Root (1963) reported 2 families, one of which revealed hydrocephalic male offspring from 2 different fathers. Warren, Lu, and Ziering (1963) reviewed a family with 3 known hydrocephalic brothers and 2 additional probable hydrocephalic males. Abdul-Karin, Iliya, and Iskandar (1964) reported 3 consecutive stillborn hydrocephalics from a single mother. Williamson (1965) discussed one family with 2 hydrocephalic brothers and another family with a male hydrocephalic, whose mother had one hydrocephalic brother and another brother with probable hydrocephalus. An additional 2 families were described by Walker (1960), one with 4 hydrocephalic males.

The evidence that the families reported demonstrate an X-linked recessive inheritance pattern was as follows: hydrocephalus occurred only in males; all females were normal; the condition was transmitted from one generation to another by a carrier female; and finally, the reports of Edwards *et al.* (1961), Needleman and Root (1963), and Walker (1960), in which a woman had hydrocephalic male offspring from two different fathers. The purpose of this paper is to present a family with X-linked inherited hydrocephalus in which 4 males were affected in 2 generations. The importance of distinguishing this group of patients from non-familial hydrocephalus and the relation of genetic counselling will be discussed.

Case Report

The propositus (Pedigree III.2) presented at Children's Memorial Hospital at 8 days of age with an enlarged head and probable congenital megacolon. He was the product of a full-term uncomplicated pregnancy of a gravida 2 para 2, 25-year-old woman whose previous child, a female infant with 18-trisomy, died at 17 months of age. Delivery was complicated by the large head, and forceps were necessary. Head circumference at birth was 41·0 cm., weight 3643 g., chest circumference 31·5 cm., and anterior and posterior fontanelles both measured 3 × 4 cm. The head did not transilluminate and skull x-rays showed no calcifications.

The head circumference on the fifth day after admission was 41·5 cm., and ventriculograms revealed symmetrical dilatation of both lateral ventricles, normal third ventricle, and no visualization of air beyond the proximal portion of the aqueduct of Sylvius, the post-operative diagnosis being stenosis of the aqueduct. A ventriculo-atrial shunt was performed on the 21st hospital day, at which time the head circumference was 42·5 cm. Subsequent pneumoencephalograms and Pantopaque studies further substantiated the diagnosis of a blockage of the aqueduct of Sylvius at the junction of the lower two-thirds with the upper two-thirds of the aqueduct.

Chromosome studies on the propositus and his mother yielded the following results: propositus 46XY, mother 46XX, with no chromosomal abnormalities observed in either case.

A male maternal cousin (Pedigree III.4) of the propositus was brought to Children's Memorial Hospital at 3 years of age with a previous diagnosis of hydrocephalus and mental retardation. Physical examination on admission revealed a head circumference of 55 cm. An operative pneumoventriculogram and Pantopaque ventriculogram demonstrated dilatation of the lateral ventricles, an enlarged third ventricle, and aqueductal stenosis. A III–IV ventriculo-ventriculostomy was carried out at a later date. Two male sibs of this cousin are normal.

184

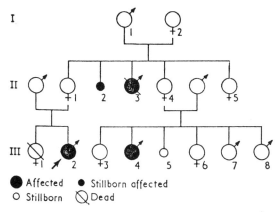

● Affected   ● Stillborn affected
○ Stillborn   ◐ Dead

Fig. Pedigree of the family with X-linked hydrocephalus. There are 4 affected members (darkened symbols), one of whom was an affected stillborn male (II.2).

Two maternal uncles of the propositus were also known to be hydrocephalic, one a stillborn (Pedigree II.2), and the other (Pedigree II.3) dying at the age of 11: in this case, an aqueductal stenosis was found at necropsy. Further investigation of the family history revealed no other instances of hydrocephalus.

Discussion

Many surveys have been carried out in recent years to determine the incidence of hydrocephalus and other central nervous system abnormalities (Table). The incidence of congenital hydrocephalus, not associated with myelomeningocele, varies from 0·22 per thousand live births to 1·8 per thousand total births. Carter (1963) has estimated the incidence in Europe to be approximately 0·5 per

TABLE
STUDIES OF MAJOR CONGENITAL MALFORMATIONS

Author	Location of Study	No. of Cases	Incidence of Congenital Hydrocephalus (per 1000 total births)
Williamson (1965)	Southampton	14,907	0·90
Wallace, Baumgartner, and Rich (1953)	New York	1501	0·22★
Book (1951)	Sweden	44,109	1·00
McIntosh et al. (1954)	New York City	5739	0·90†
Neel (1958)	Japan	64,569	0·30
Pleydell (1960)	Northamptonshire	60,890	0·60★
McKeown and Record (1960)	Birmingham	56,760	1·80
McDonald (1961)	Watford and St. Albans	3179	1·60
Simpkiss and Lowe (1961)	Kampala	2068	1·50

★ Per thousand live births.
† Per thousand deliveries.

185

thousand births. It appears that the vast majority of cases of hydrocephalus are not primarily of genetic origin. If one combines the studies of Penrose (1960), McKeown and Record (1960), and MacMahon, Pugh, and Ingalls (1953), in which sibs of a propositus with hydrocephalus were studied, only one hydrocephalic infant was found in the 200 cases studied. In addition, analysis of the data of Record (1959, personal communication by Edwards et al. (1961)), showed no affected male sib of 50 male propositi studied.

The true incidence of aqueductal stenosis is not known, but among 44 necropsies of cases with infantile hydrocephalus, Elvidge (1966) found 30% with aqueductal stenosis. It is of interest that in our cases as well as in 5 others (Bickers and Adams, 1949; Edwards et al., 1961; Needleman and Root, 1963; Warren et al., 1963) previously studied, the pathological lesion producing the hydrocephalus was aqueductal stenosis.

Though estimates of the incidence of X-linked hydrocephalus are about 2% (Brit. med. J., 1962) of all cases of uncomplicated hydrocephalus, every effort should be made to recognize this group of patients. While the over-all recurrence risk appears to be of the order of 0·5 to 1%, in these X-linked cases the recurrence risk will usually be higher. Where the mother is known, from the family history, to be a carrier, it will be 50% for later brothers, and though none of the daughters will be affected 50% will in turn be carriers. Since there is no way to recognize the carrier state, one should exercise care in counselling parents of hydrocephalic offspring. Probably the greatest caution should be exercised when aqueductal stenosis is found in a male propositus.

Summary

A family showing the syndrome of X-linked inherited hydrocephalus with 4 affected members in 2 generations is presented. The combined incidence of all forms of uncomplicated congenital hydrocephalus is reviewed and compared with the incidence to be expected in the X-linked form. The relevance of these figures to genetic counselling is discussed.

The authors wish to thank Dr. Michael Jerva for allowing them to study his patient, and Regina Kavaliunas for help in interviewing the family.

Supported in part by grants from the U.S. Public Health Service (1-S01-FR-5370-04).

186

REFERENCES

Abdul-Karin, R., Iliya, F., and Iskandar, G. (1964). Consecutive hydrocephalus: Report of 2 cases. *Obstet. and Gynec.*, **24**, 376.

Bamatter, F. (1949). Acquisitions récentes concernant les hydrocéphalies inflammatoires chez l'enfant. Travail d'habilitation de la faculté de Medicine de Genève (dactylographie) 87. (Quoted by Edwards and by Borle.)

Bickers, D. S., and Adams, R. D. (1949). Hereditary stenosis of the aqueduct of Sylvius as a cause of congenital hydrocephalus. *Brain*, **72**, 246.

Book, J. A. (1951). The incidence of congenital diseases and defects in a South Swedish population. *Acta genet (Basel)*, **2**, 289.

Borle, A. (1953). Sur l'étiologie de l'hydrocéphalie congénitale. A propos d'un case d'hydrocéphalie concordante chez des jumeaux univitellins. *J. Génét. hum.*, **2**, 157.

Brit. med. J. (1962). Editorial. Sex-linked hydrocephalus with severe mental defect. **1**, 168.

Carter, C. O. (1963). Incidence and aetiology (of congenital malformation in childhood). *In Congenital Abnormalities in Infancy*, p. 1. Ed. by A. P. Norman. Blackwell Scientific Publications, Oxford.

Edwards, J. H. (1961). The syndrome of sex-linked hydrocephalus. *Arch. Dis. Childh.*, **36**, 486.

——, Norman, R. M., and Roberts, J. M. (1961). Sex-linked hydrocephalus: Report of a family with 15 affected members. *ibid.*, **36**, 481.

Elvidge, A. R. (1966). Treatment of obstructive lesions of the aqueduct of Sylvius and the fourth ventricle by interventriculostomy. *J. Neurosurg.*, **24**, 11.

Gellman, V. (1959). Congenital hydrocephalus in monovular twins. *Arch. Dis. Childh.*, **34**, 274.

McDonald, A. D. (1961). Matronal health in early pregnancy and congenital defect; final report on a prospective inquiry. *Brit. J. prev. soc. Med.*, **15**, 154.

McIntosh, R., Merritt, K. K., Richards, M. R., Samuels, M. H., and Bellows, M. T. (1954). The incidence of congenital malformations: A study of 5,964 pregnancies. *Pediatrics*, **14**, 505.

McKeown, T., and Record, R. G. (1960). Malformations in a population observed for five years after birth. In *Ciba Foundation Symposium on Congenital Malformations*, p. 2 Ed. by G. E. W. Wolstenholme and C. M. O'Connor. Churchill, London.

MacMahon, B., Pugh, T. F., and Ingalls, T. H. (1953). Anencephalus, spina bifida, and hydrocephalus: Incidence related to sex, race, and season of birth, and incidence in siblings. *Brit. J. prev. soc. Med.*, **7**, 211.

Needleman, H. L., and Root, A. W. (1963). Sex-linked hydrocephalus: Report of two families, with chromosomal study of two cases. *Pediatrics*, **31**, 396.

Neel, J. V. (1958). A study of major congenital defects in Japanese infants. *Amer. J. hum. Genet.*, **10**, 398.

Penrose, L. S. (1960). Genetic causes of malformations. In *Ciba Foundation Symposium on Congenital Malformations*, p. 22. Ed. by G. E. W. Wolstenholme and C. M. O'Connor. Churchill, London.

Pleydell, M. J. (1960). Anencephaly and other congenital abnormalities. An epidemiological study in Northamptonshire. *Brit. med. J.*, **1**, 309.

Simpkiss, M., and Lowe, A. (1961). Congenital abnormalities in the African newborn. *Arch. Dis. Childh.*, **36**, 404.

Walker, J. (1960). Discussion, genetical causes of malformations and the search for their origins. In *Ciba Foundation Symposium on Congenital Malformations*, p. 30. Ed. by G. E. W. Wolstenholme and C. M. O'Connor. Churchill, London.

Wallace, H. M., Baumgartner, L., and Rich, H. (1953). Congenital malformations and birth injuries in New York City. *Pediatrics*, **12**, 525.

Warren, M. C., Lu, A. T., and Ziering, W. H. (1963). Sex-linked hydrocephalus with aqueductal stenosis. *J. Pediat.*, **63**, 1104.

Williamson, E. M. (1965). Incidence and family aggregation of major congenital malformations of central nervous system. *J. med. Genet.*, **2**, 161.

Zimmer, K. (1952). Uber familiäres Auftreten von Hydrozephalus. *Geburtsh. u. Frauenheilk.*, **12**, 447.

187

Cartilage–Hair Hypoplasia

A Rare and Recessive Cause of Dwarfism

R. B. LOWRY, M.B., B.Ch., F.R.C.P.(C.),

J. A. BIRKBECK, M.B., Ch.B.,

P. H. PADWICK, M.B., B.Ch.

BETTY J. WOOD, M.D.

CARTILAGE–HAIR hypoplasia was first delineated by McKusick *et al.*[1] following genetic studies in the Amish, a population isolate in the United States This sect originated in the canton of Berne, Switzerland, in 1693 and began emigrating to North America in the 1700's. Their language is a South German dialect.

As the designation implies, a cartilage deficiency at the growing ends of the bones causes a short-limbed, disproportionate type of dwarf along with a sparse growth of fine hair. Since McKusick's report other cases among the non-Amish have been recognized (Maroteaux *et al.*;[2] Irwin;[3] Beals[4]).

Many cases of short-limbed dwarfism are mistakenly labeled achondroplasia. The medical and psychologic management of such cases does not differ from cartilage–hair hypoplasia, but the genetic counseling is different. When normal parents have a baby with true achondroplasia this is probably the result of a new dominant mutation and thus the recurrence risk is zero. In contrast, in cartilage–hair hypoplasia the recurrence risk is high (25 per cent) since it is due to a recessive gene.

Description of Case

L. O. is the eldest child of healthy unrelated German parents who are of normal stature. She was born after a full-term pregnancy and normal delivery. Birth weight was 3.9 Kg. During pregnancy there were no unusual events or drugs taken. The first few years of her life were notable for repeated attacks of otitis media and mastoiditis for which a mastoidectomy was performed. An attack of chickenpox was unusually severe and left a large number of scars.

She was first studied for short stature when she was four years old but no definite diagnosis was reached. She was restudied in 1968 at ten years old when the present diagnosis was made. Her height then was 111 cm. (height age: five years, two months) (Fig. 1). Her lower segment was 52 cm. and span, 110.5 cm. Her hair was blonde, short, extremely fine and silky. The skull was normal in shape and size. Numerous small pigmented nevi were scattered over the upper trunk and back. The fingers were short and hyperextensible; the nails were normal. Many other joints, including the elbow, could be hyperextended. The lateral malleolus was significantly lower than the medial, reflecting increased fibular length. The secondary teeth were fully erupted and were normal. The remaining systems disclosed no abnormality. Intelligence was normal.

Laboratory Studies

Hemoglobin, 15.1 Gm./100 ml.; WBC, 4,700 per cu. mm.; polymorphs, 57; staff cells, six; lymphocytes, 28; monocytes, eight; basophils, one. Serum electrolytes, BUN, protein electrophoresis, immune globulins, calcium, phosphate, alkaline phosphatase and protein-bound iodine were normal. Buccal smear was chromatin positive and she had a normal female karyotype. Plasma growth hormone responses to infusions of insulin and arginine were normal. Microscopic examination of the stool revealed a few fat droplets. Assay of stool showed 510 μg. trypsin per Gm. and 810 μg. chymotrypsin per Gm.—both within normal limits. Radiologic studies disclosed thickening and irregularity at the metaphyses of all long bones particularly the radius, femur and tibia (Fig. 2). These were consistent with the radiologic diagnosis of metaphyseal dysostosis.

Leukocyte counts were performed every five days for six weeks to exclude the possibility of

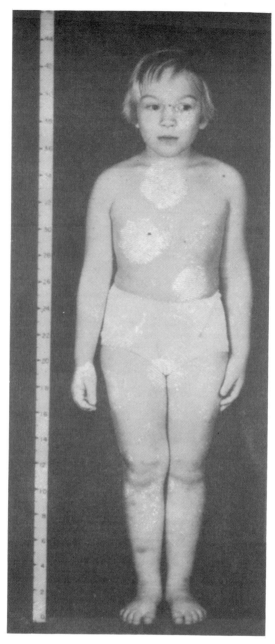

Fig. 1. Patient at ten years old. Her height is only
111 cm. (44-1/2 inches).

190

cyclic neutropenia. The majority of the observations were around 5,000/cu. mm., with a range of 3,600 to 10,000—all differential counts were within the normal range.

Microscopic examination of her scalp hair revealed an extremely thin caliber without a pigment core. Tensile strength and amino-acid content of her hair were studied, with results to be reported elsewhere (Coupe et al.[5]). Because of her dwarfism, the patient became increasingly withdrawn and it was decided not to pursue any further investigation despite the good rapport established with her and her family.

The three younger siblings, males, were all about the 50th percentile in height, had hyperextensible elbow joints, and two could hyperextend their fingers. One of these two had fine, thin hair whose caliber was between that of the patient and of the other two siblings.

Discussion

Although there are some differences on physical examination between our patient and those described by McKusick we believe that there is no reason to doubt the diagnosis. The hair is sparse and fine. Our patient could hyperextend her elbows whereas McKusick described an inability to fully extend this joint. Some of his patients had malabsorption, whereas our patient did not have such symptoms and stool enzymes and stool microscopy were normal in screening tests.

Burke et al.[6] have described an association between metaphyseal dysostosis, pancreatic exocrine deficiency with malabsorption, and neutropenia. However, their patients were not reported as having short stature or fine, sparse hair so that this association remains unexplained. We were not able to prove the existence of cyclic neutropenia in our child. A low normal leukocyte count also was noted in the patient of Beals.[4]

Chickenpox appears to cause unusually severe upsets in children with cartilage–hair hypoplasia. This feature was found in the Amish patients as well as our own. Burgert et al.[7] described a patient who in most respects had

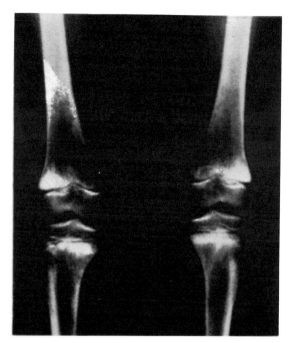

Fig. 2. X-ray of knees. Note irregular sclerotic
appearance along the metaphyseal edge.

symptoms similar to cartilage–hair hypoplasia.
However, her hair was thought not to be as
sparse and in addition she showed extreme
hyperphosphatasia.

McKusick demonstrated in bone biopsy an
inadequacy of cartilage in this condition.
Thus there is no specific therapy available
for the dwarfism. We feel that families should
not be dismissed with this information but
rather that they should be supported and
counseled over a long period. The psychologic
problems of dwarfism in general, as surveyed
recently by Drash,[8] provide some guidance for
the physician in how to handle the problems
of withdrawal, immaturity, underachievement
at school and parental denial.

Since cartilage–hair hypoplasia appears due
to homozygosity for an autosomal recessive
gene, genetic counseling becomes extremely

important. McKusick says that there may be incomplete penetrance of the gene if dwarfism is taken as the phenotype, and that some individuals with abnormally thin hair in these families may be homozygotes.

There may be some sex influences in the penetrance of the gene since he found a disproportionate number of female cases. However, one brother of our patient has fine hair and thus possibly may be a homozygote. Incomplete penetrance may reduce the recurrence risk from 25 per cent to somewhere around 20 per cent. We feel that parents should have this information to make an informed decision about future pregnancies. Probably few families would choose to accept a recurrence risk greater than 15 per cent, particularly since the adult height seems to be less than 150 cm., with a range in McKusick's cases from 108.5 to 148.6 cm.

Although the parents of our patients were not of the Amish community, they were both born in Germany. McKusick has suggested that the gene probably existed in Europe prior to the migration of the Amish to North America.

Acknowledgment

This study was supported by National Health grant (Canada) 609-7-155 and by the Children's Hospital, Vancouver. The authors thank Dr. Margaret J. Corey for the chromosome analysis and Dr. James R. Miller for reviewing the manuscript.

References

1. McKusick, V. A., Eldridge, R., Hostetler, J. A., Ruangwit, U. and Egeland, J. A.: Dwarfism in the Amish; II. cartilage-hair hypoplasia. Bul. Hopkins Hosp. 116: 285, 1965.
2. Maroteaux, P., Savart, P., Lefebvre, J. and Royer, P.: Les formes partielles de la dysostose métaphysaire. Presse Med. 71: 1523, 1963.
3. Irwin, G. A. L.: Cartilage-hair hypoplasia (CHH) variant of familial metaphyseal dysostosis. Radiology 86: 926, 1966.
4. Beals, R. K.: Cartilage-hair hypoplasia. J. Bone Joint Surg. 50-A: 1245, 1968.
5. Coupe, R.: Personal communication, 1969.

6. Burke, V., Colebatch, J. H., Anderson, C. M. and Simons, M. J.: Association of pancreatic insufficiency and chronic neutropenia in childhood. Arch. Dis. Child. **42:** 147, 1967.
7. Burgert, E. O., Dower, J. C. and Tauxe, W. N.: A new syndrome; regenerative anemia, malabsorption (celiac), dyschondroplasia and hyperphosphatemia. J. Pediat. **67:** 711, 1965.
8. Drash, P. W.: Psychologic counseling; dwarfism. *In* Endocrine and Genetic Diseases of Childhood, L. I. Gardner, ed. Philadelphia, W. B. Saunders, 1968, p. 1014.

194

AUTHOR INDEX